Lisa,
Thanks for all
your help and support
this year. From your
friends at
White O'Connor

yoganap

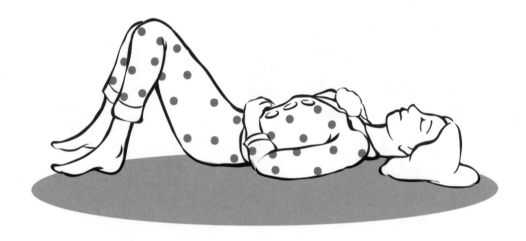

yoganap

RESTORATIVE POSES
FOR DEEP RELAXATION

Kristen Rentz

illustrations by Kajiah Jacobs

MARLOWE & COMPANY
NEW YORK

YOGANAP: *Restorative Poses for Deep Relaxation*
Copyright © 2005 by Kristen Rentz
Illustrations by Kajiah Jacobs

Published by
Marlowe & Company
An Imprint of Avalon Publishing Group Incorporated
245 West 17th Street • 11th Floor
New York, NY 10011-5300

AVALON

Library of Congress Cataloging-in-Publication Data

Rentz, Kristen, 1975-
Yoganap : restorative poses for deep relaxation / Kristen Rentz ; illustrations by Kajiah Jacobs.
  p. cm.
ISBN: 1-56924-350-6 (pbk.)
1. Hatha yoga. 2. Relaxation. I. Title.
RA781.7.R46 2005
613.7'046—dc22
2005012030

ISBN-13: 978-1-56924-350-3

9 8 7 6 5 4 3 2 1

DESIGNED BY PAULINE NEUWIRTH, NEUWIRTH & ASSOCIATES, INC.

Printed in Canada

for
owen matthew lewis

acknowledgments

I CREDIT THIS BOOK to my teachers. Among my greatest teachers are plants, classic literature, cats, joy, and genuine suffering. In addition, I would like to express profound gratitude to my human teachers:

B. K. S. Iyengar for pioneering and developing the poses that form the foundation for restorative yoga.

Chris Stein for leading my first restorative yoga class and opening my heart to this practice, as well as Judith Lasater, who sparked my desire to teach others the power of deep relaxation.

Maty Ezraty and Chuck Miller for creating YogaWorks, my yoga home.

My friend and illustrator, Kajiah Jacobs, for displaying endless patience and creativity.

My agent, Jeff Herman, for his vast experience and for believing in *YogaNap*.

My publisher, Matthew Lore, for giving me this opportunity, and my editor, Kylie Foxx, for her editorial expertise.

My students for inspiring me to continue to grow as a teacher. The trust and expressed appreciation of Ben Wong, Jane Margolis, and Richard Ford never ceases to amaze me.

My friends and colleagues for believing in me. Jessica Berger Gross, my great friend and fellow writer and yoga teacher, for responding to several dozen e-mails every week. Michele Bickley for sharing her experience, faith, and love. Meredith Blake for her guidance, support, and strength. Sonya Cottle for teaching me how to be a true friend.

My family for giving me the space to become myself. My mom and dad for trusting me and having faith. My sister Dani for her care and comfort throughout my life. My sister Heather for her creativity and individuality. My niece and nephew Sophie and Max for showing me the depth of my capacity to love.

Joanna Poppink for giving me a new lens through which to see, providing a container in which I could safely develop, a garden in which I could watch life happen, and for teaching me the power of fairy tales, myths, and dreams.

Owen Lewis, my love, for grounding me, loving me unconditionally, surprising me daily with his insight, making me smile from the inside out, and keeping me company during Saturday morning writing sessions.

contents

2 **yoga**vitaminc ✳ 30
poses to boost your immune system

3 **yoga**alarmclock ✳ 52
poses to invigorate your body and mind

4 **yogalullaby** ✳ 72
poses to cure your insomnia

7 **yoga**headache**rx** ✳ 134
poses for headache relief

8 **yoga**break ✳ 156

poses to relax at work or on the go

ARE YOU STRESSED? Overworked? Overtired? Feel like you need a nap? You're not alone. We're all running out of steam! What we desperately need is a YogaNap. Taking a YogaNap is the simple stress solution, the anxiety antidote, the cure for common craziness. While taking a YogaNap, you'll mostly practice what are called restorative yoga poses. I discovered restorative yoga a few years into my personal yoga practice. A vigorous yoga practice had certainly helped me cope with the stress of law school—so much so that I was practicing six days a week. I was healthy and strong, but I was exhausted. One day, I found myself struggling to decide between going to yoga and going home to take a nap. Without thinking, the phrase flew out of my mouth—I need a YogaNap. At that moment, a light bulb went off and I decided to incorporate more restorative yoga into my life. It worked! I was stronger and had more energy than ever. I noticed,

introduction

however, that there were very few restorative yoga classes, even in Los Angeles. YogaNap grew out of my desire to share the amazing effect that restorative yoga has had on my life. I have not only used the techniques presented in YogaNap to stay calm as I juggle my two careers—as a litigation attorney and a yoga teacher—but I have also watched my students' lives transform through working with these postures.

Restorative yoga truly does provide the key element to managing chronic stress—deep, thorough relaxation. This comfortable, nurturing, restful practice is even more restful than taking a nap, because even during sleep, the mind is still very active. While taking a YogaNap, the mind becomes as calm and soothed as the body, while the nervous system comes into complete balance. Regardless of age, fitness level, or flexibility, nearly anyone can practice restorative yoga. No longer do we have to endure the immense pressures of daily stress wishing there was a solution. There is! Take a YogaNap today.

what, exactly, is restorative yoga?

Your mom has a mat rolled up in the back of her car, your coworkers are replacing power lunches with power yoga classes, celebrities are toting designer mat bags—there's airplane yoga, hot yoga, hypnoyoga, and even doggie yoga. But is all this yoga doing the trick? Many of us turn to yoga to relieve stress, but often our yoga is as fast paced and rushed as our lives. Getting better at anything takes practice, so we have to practice relaxing and slowing down. That is exactly what restorative yoga provides—optimal conditions created by placing and holding our bodies in supported, relaxing postures, so that we can really learn to let go, quiet and calm our racing minds, and soothe our tense and clenching muscles.

Stress exists not only in the mind, but in the physical body as well. When we start to relax and release our bodies, our minds have the opportunity to follow. Think of a crying, restless baby. To soothe the baby, the adult picks up the baby, holds the baby, rocks the baby, and gradually the baby's sobbing slows, the tightness in the baby's face disappears, and the baby is once again peaceful and serene. As adults, we can re-create the same sense of being held and feeling supported and safe with restorative yoga. Restorative yoga helps "restore" a sense of balance, peace, and well being—physically and emotionally.

YogaNap provides a fun, easy, accessible way to learn and practice restorative yoga. In *YogaNap*, you'll use a variety of props like blankets, bolsters, straps, and blocks to completely support the body in a variety of poses. (These props will be covered in greater detail on page 9.) You'll hold many of the poses for a couple of minutes or longer. Some of the postures provide passive stretching and stimulate different areas of the body. Others are designed simply to allow pure, unqualified rest.

holding up vs. letting go

Much, if not all of our days are spent "holding ourselves up." We physically hold ourselves up with our muscles and bones, and we emotionally hold ourselves up with a variety of coping mechanisms. And for good reason—we have lives to live, things to accomplish, and people counting on us. We wear a "social mask," facing the world with an acceptable neutral or even guarded expression, often not even recognizing our own feelings. In fact, we get so good at holding ourselves up that it becomes difficult to let go and relax. Even when we allow ourselves downtime or breaks, we have trouble accessing our emotions, we resist experiencing vulnerability, and we certainly struggle to relax. We need to relearn how to let go and let ourselves be held. We can encourage this process by relying on the physical support of props, sending the message to our nervous system that it is safe to let go, just as being held calms a crying baby. Slowly, over time, it will become easier and easier to let go, and we'll be able to tap into this ability throughout our days, whenever tension mounts.

Letting go requires conscious awareness; it doesn't happen automatically. In each and every YogaNap pose, we must continue to direct and focus our attention to the process of letting go. It's often helpful to use visualization. We can imagine that our entire body is melting, as we soften the facial muscles and relax the tongue into the back of the throat, feeling as though the skin is sliding off the bone. We can envision ourselves being held in the palm of a giant hand. We can even see ourselves lying on the belly of a giant breathing bear, or picture ourselves engulfed in benevolent, warm light. If you continue to work with soothing, enveloping images, you'll find something that resonates with you.

The importance of long, smooth, clear breathing cannot be understated. When we allow ourselves to breathe deeply, we automatically slow down. Remember the restless baby—as the baby's sobbing subsides, the baby's breathing slows. As we completely fill our lungs with cleansing air, we feel more connected and present in our bodies, we get in touch with our feelings, and since we are supported in our restorative pose, we are able to surrender some of our tightness and tension. Breathe in and out through your nose, working to match the length of your inhale to the length of your exhale. Sense the rhythm in your breath, and work to make each breath a little bit longer and smoother than the one before it. You'll notice each breath carries away a little bit of stress, just as a river over time smoothes a rock. Keep breathing, learn to respect relaxation as a gradual process, and you'll be greatly rewarded with an inner sense of strength and resilience.

Using conscious breathing and visualization will also help us let go of the incessant mental chatter that can keep us on edge. Adding a mantra or a repetitive phrase to your breathing can help draw your attention away from your thoughts and onto your breath. A mantra can be as simple as repeating the word "let" to yourself as you inhale, and the word "go" to yourself as you exhale. Again, experiment— find a mantra that works for you, remain open to using different words depending on your mood. You may even try adding a "color" to your breath, inhaling a soothing color, and exhaling a color you associate with tension and negativity.

achieving balance

Practicing conscious relaxation with restorative yoga poses will help restore your natural sense of physical, mental, and emotional equilibrium. As you continue to work with the *YogaNap* techniques, you'll become increasingly aware of areas in which you feel out of balance. On any given day, you may feel excessive anger, you may feel lethargic, you may feel excited, you may feel sad—you'll likely experience many feelings all at once. Setting an intention for your practice of yoga can be extremely helpful in restoring balance to your system. A great way to arrive at an intention is to identify where you are feeling *out* of balance, and set as an intention the opposite energy. For example, if you are feeling angry, you might choose to devote your practice to cultivating compassion or forgiveness; if you are feeling emotionally heavy, you may add a sense of lightness to your practice. Remind yourself of your intention throughout your practice, perhaps bringing your intention into the rest of your day or week.

the poses

The poses can be broken down into five general categories: forward bends, back bends, twists, inversions, and hip openers. Each type of pose targets a specific area of the body and fosters a particular energetic quality. Forward bends work to release the lower back and are very quieting for the mind. Back bends, in contrast, are very energizing; they open the chest and stimulate the spine. Twists work to wring out the internal organs, freeing up stagnant energy. Inversions, or any pose in which the hips are more elevated than the head, affect hormone levels and balance the lymphatic system. Hip openers restore healthy movement in the hip joints and provide a sense of freedom.

As you continue to practice the techniques described in this book, you'll begin to see how different poses help create different physical and emotional states. Each chapter highlights a common way we can fall out of balance and offers poses to restore balance. You are encouraged to follow the provided sequences; as you become more comfortable with the postures, you can begin to create your own sequences. Create your own sequences based on how your body responds to the particular poses—just as you crave certain foods, you'll find yourself craving certain poses. Allow yourself the freedom to listen to your body and explore combining poses accordingly.

Although it's not imperative that you complete the poses in an entire chapter—you can mix and match poses—you should always finish with a very passive resting pose (examples of which close each chapter), which you should hold for at least 5 minutes. And while this book focuses on restful, restorative yoga, not every pose is completely passive, though many of them are. Some of the poses will seem precarious at first. Give yourself time, be patient, allow yourself to be a beginner—

remember, you are learning a whole new way of being. Begin by holding each pose for the minimum amount of time, and work up gradually to a longer duration.

Our bodies are alive, unique, and constantly changing—not every pose is appropriate for every *body*, and not every pose is appropriate for every *day*. Listen to your body, and never attempt a pose that doesn't feel right or strains your body in any way. Remember that some days your body may feel very open and limber, and other days it may feel as stiff as a board. Rather than judging these fluctuations, respect them, and practice in a way that nurtures your body and spirit as they are on any given day. There is no "right" or "wrong" way to do a pose. Use comfort as your barometer, and keep in mind that pain is never good. When moving in and out of poses, move slowly and carefully, and especially after a long hold, think about your exit movements before you ease into them, so as to avoid any abrupt impact on your nervous system.

what are props, and how do i use them?

The *YogaNap* poses rely upon a variety of props to help create the feeling of being held and supported. We position blankets, blocks, and bolsters in different shapes and then climb on top and let go. At times we use straps of various lengths to secure our arms, legs, or bodies so we won't have to make an effort to hold ourselves up and can instead focus on—you guessed it—letting go. We'll be placing the props in a variety of shapes, but we'll be using the following "building block shapes" repeatedly in several poses

props and prop formations

Don't be intimidated by the props! They're here to help! And you certainly don't have to use professional yoga props. You can substitute many household items for traditional yoga props. You can use blankets, pillows, towels, and couch cushions for blankets and bolsters; books instead of blocks; and belts and scarves in lieu of straps. Be creative—a bag of rice makes a great eye pillow! Sometimes the best props are the floor and the wall. And by all means, don't be stingy with the props—strip your beds, empty your closets—add props to any pose. Make yourself comfortable—use as many props as you need to in order to feel fully supported. Experimentation is encouraged—there's more than one way to fold a blanket!

If you do choose to use traditional yoga props, here's a word on placing traditional yoga straps into a looped formation: be patient—it's more complicated than it may seem. Diffuse the drama by playing with your strap until you figure out how to connect it so that the size of the loop holds tight and doesn't slip. Keep reminding yourself that the object of restorative yoga is to fully support the body so that the mind and nervous system can relax.

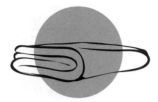

blanket
—either a traditional "yoga" blanket or any substitute that is nonquilted and approximately 8' x 10'

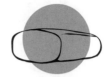

bolster
—either a traditional "yoga" bolster or any substitute that is approximately 26" x 12" x 6"

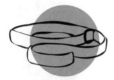

strap
—either a traditional "yoga" strap or any substitute approximately 6' long

eye pillow

block
—either a traditional "yoga" block or any substitute that is approximately 6" x 4" x 9"

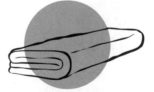

long-folded blanket
—Fold a blanket to create an approximately 30" x 10" x 3" rectangle.

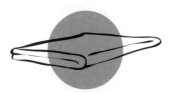

open-folded blanket
—Fold a blanket to create an approximately
30" x 20" x 1½" rectangle.

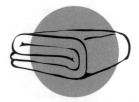

square-folded blanket
—Fold a blanket to create an
approximately 20" x 15" x 3" square.

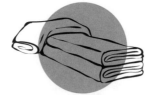

t-formation
—Place 2 long-folded blankets on top of each
other. Cross a third long-folded blanket across
the blankets to form a T shape.

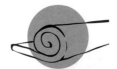

thick-rolled blanket
—Roll a blanket into a short, thick
tube with an approximately
10" diameter.

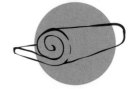

thin-rolled blanket
—Roll a blanket into a long tube with
an approximately 5" diameter.

helpful hints, considerations, and recommendations

❋ Consider using an eye pillow, perhaps even one that is scented with soothing lavender, in the more passive poses—the gentle pressure on your eyes will feel wonderful.

❋ Wear comfortable, loose-fitting clothing, and if your feet are cold, wear socks! It's very difficult to relax when you are cold.

❋ Allow yourself to give in completely to the support of the props—doing so will greatly enhance your experience.

❋ Use a small timer with a nonjarring alarm to time your poses so that you don't have to watch the clock.

❋ Consciously relax your mind in every pose, continuing to work on letting go of mental chatter.

❋ Take advantage of spare moments, sneak in mini YogaNaps throughout the day.

❋ As often as you remember, take a deep breath.

❋ Look for a restorative yoga class in your area, find a teacher that makes you feel safe.

❋ As with any physical exercise program, consult your health professional before you begin.

❋ Create a special place and time for your YogaNap. Clear some space near a wall where you know you won't be disturbed. Practice on a soft carpet or lay a blanket or mat down for comfort in every pose.

theposes

1

IF ONLY THERE were another hour, or two hours, or ten hours in the day.... We like to think it would make a difference, but would it? Inevitably, more tasks and chores, more responsibilities and demands would swoop right in to fill the time, and we'd be right back in the frazzled state where we started. The undeniable truth is that if we are going to thrive instead of merely survive in our often crazy, fast-paced lives, we have to learn to prioritize. Interestingly enough, when we make time for ourselves, stop to take a breath, and choose to slow down while others are speeding up, we actually conserve our energy, become more efficient, and have more time!

In each of the YogaAahhh poses in this chapter, the body is fully supported with props, in order to create a feeling of being held. This allows the nervous system to still and the body and mind to fully and deeply relax. When accompanied with slow, steady, mindful breathing, these poses truly provide a remedy for chronic stress.

It may be counterintuitive, but when you choose to take time for yourself, when you choose to make your physical and mental health a priority, when you practice these poses regularly—even once a week—you'll start to move a little slower, you'll be calmer and more compassionate, and you'll notice that you have more time for the things that matter most to you … YogaAahhh!

* **child's pose on blankets**

* **super-supported bridge pose**

* **floating body rest**

* **comfy angle rest**

* **cozy blanket twist**

* **legs-up-the-wall cocoon**

* **super-supported resting pose**

child's pose on blankets

CHILD'S POSE ON BLANKETS relaxes and soothes the lower back, relieves tension in the neck and shoulders, and is very emotionally comforting and grounding.

you will need: *1 to 3 long-folded blankets*

* Kneel on the floor with your knees apart, sitting on your heels, with your big toes touching.

* Stack one, two, or three long-folded blankets between your legs. Stack the blankets high enough so that when you fold forward, you can relax onto them completely without holding yourself up at all.

* Gently fold your torso over onto the blankets, resting your head to one side. Halfway through your hold, turn your head to the other side for an even neck stretch.

* Find a comfortable position for your arms, either alongside your body or in front of you.

* Close your eyes, let go, and breathe, holding each side for 1 to 5 minutes.

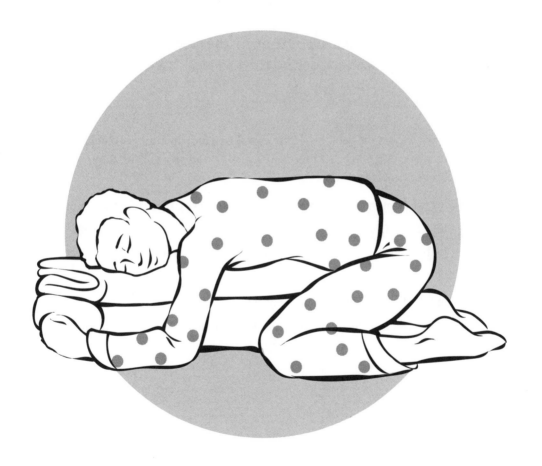

super-supported bridge pose

SUPER-SUPPORTED BRIDGE POSE opens the heart, allowing deep, clear breathing while soothing aching feet and legs.

you will need: *4 bolsters or 8 long-folded blankets, 3 straps, thin-rolled blanket*

✳ Stack two sets of two bolsters (or two sets of four long-folded blankets—a total of eight) end to end. For stability, it's a good idea to strap the blankets/bolsters together.

✳ Place a tightened strap around your thighs to keep them together snugly.

✳ Lie on top of the props with only your head and shoulders off of the blankets resting on the floor. Place a thin rolled blanket under your neck for support.

✳ Bring the backs of your hands to rest on either side of your head.

✳ Close your eyes, let go, and breathe, holding the pose for 3 to 8 minutes.

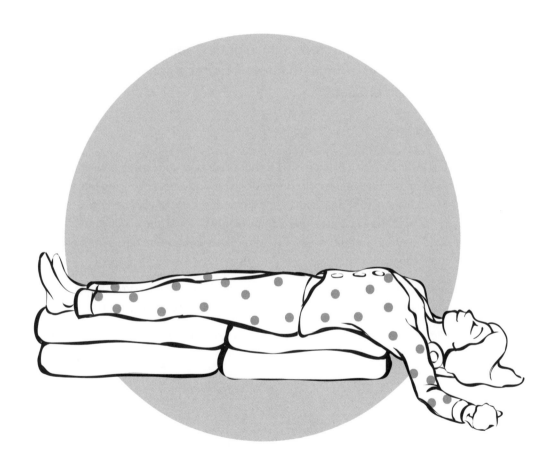

floating body rest

FLOATING BODY REST creates a weightless feeling in the body as though floating on a raft in the ocean, encouraging relaxation and a very peaceful mental state.

you will need: *1 thick-rolled blanket, 2 long-folded blankets, 1 thin-rolled blanket*

✳ Place a thick-rolled blanket on the floor to support your knees, as well as two long-folded blankets to support your middle and upper back, and one thin-rolled blanket to support your neck. The proportions of your body will determine the exact placement of the blankets—feel free to adjust them until they support the knees, middle and upper back, and neck when you are reclined.

✳ Recline on the blankets, making sure they are positioned correctly and that your arms and shoulders rest between the neck and back supports.

✳ Close your eyes, let go, and breathe for 3 to 8 minutes.

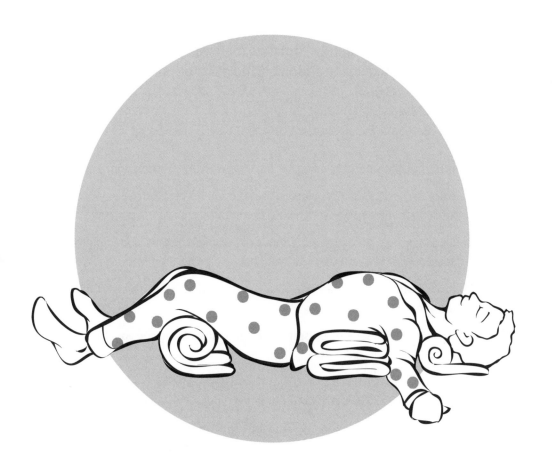

comfy angle rest

COMFY ANGLE REST gently stretches the inner thighs and hips as it increases circulation in the abdomen and eases gripping tension in the stomach and internal organs.

you will need: *3 to 5 long-folded blankets, 2 thin-rolled blankets, 3 straps, bolster (optional)*

✳ Place bolsters and/or blankets on the floor, making a T-formation.

✳ Place two long-folded blankets on the floor to support your knees and thighs and two thin-rolled blankets secured with straps to support your arms.

✳ Sit directly in front of the short end of the blankets/bolster, and bring the soles of your feet together, with your heels 12 inches from you.

✳ Place a wide looped strap over your shoulders, tightening it around your lower back and feet.

✳ Recline on the blankets/bolster, resting your arms alongside your body, palms facing the ceiling.

✳ If you experience lower back discomfort, use your hands to ease the flesh of your buttocks away from you, lengthening your lower back.

✳ Close your eyes, let go, and breathe for 3 to 10 minutes.

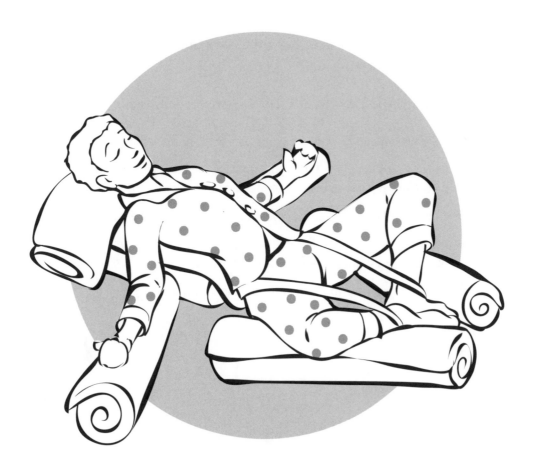

cozy blanket twist

COZY BLANKET TWIST lengthens the back and side muscles and is supremely comfortable.

you will need: *1 to 3 long-folded blankets, 2 thin-rolled blankets, bolster (optional)*

✳ Place bolster and/or blankets on the floor in a T-formation.

✳ Sit facing the top of the T, with your right hip next to the base of the T, knees bent, with your feet to the side of your left hip, heels about a foot from you.

✳ Turn toward the props, and rest your torso facedown on the base of the T.

✳ Place your arms in a comfortable position and rest your right cheek on the blanket. For a slightly deeper twist, place your left cheek on the blanket.

✳ Close your eyes, let go, and breathe for 3 to 5 minutes. Repeat on the other side.

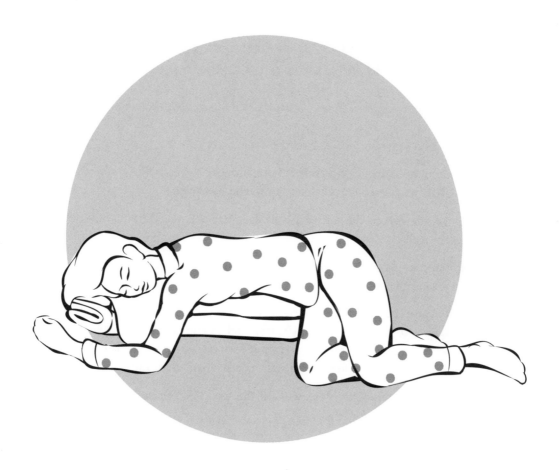

legs-up-the-wall cocoon

LEGS-UP-THE-WALL COCOON re-creates the primal comfort of being wrapped and held and takes all stress off the lower body.

you will need: *1 pair of socks, 2 to 4 long-folded blankets or 1 to 2 bolsters, 1 strap, additional blanket*

✳ Put on a pair of warm, cozy socks.

✳ Stack two to four long-folded blankets, or one to two bolsters, and place them 4 to 6 inches from the wall, running parallel to it.

✳ Sit sideways on the middle of the blankets/bolster(s), with your right side to the wall.

✳ Support yourself with your left hand as you swing your legs up the wall and recline on your back.

✳ Reverse your hands by your shoulders, so that your palms are flat on the floor with your fingers facing your shoulders, and pressing into the floor for leverage, adjust yourself so that your lower back is on the blankets/bolster, and your sit bones are resting in the space between the props and the wall.

✳ Once situated, bend your knees and tighten a strap around your shins to keep your legs together.

✳ Drape a blanket over your legs, helping to provide a cocoon for your body.

✳ Extend your legs back up the wall, bending your knees slightly if it's more comfortable for you. Make sure the strap is tight enough so that keeping your legs extended is effortless.

✳ Close your eyes, let go, and breathe for 5 to 10 minutes.

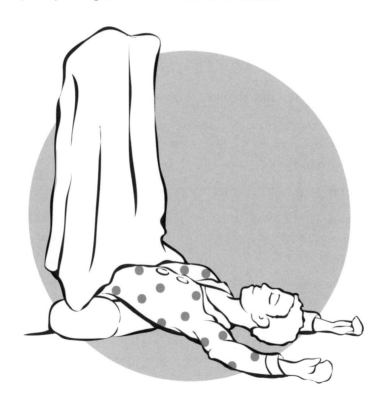

super-supported resting pose

SUPER-SUPPORTED RESTING POSE is the single most important *YogaNap* pose, providing the ultimate conditions for true, deep relaxation.

you will need: *1 pair of socks, 1 thin-rolled blanket, 1 thick-rolled blanket, 1 long-folded blanket, 1 square-folded blanket, 5 additonal blankets (optional)*

✳ Put on comfy socks for warmth.

✳ Place a thin-rolled blanket to support your ankles and a thick-rolled blanket to support your knees. The exact placement of the blankets will depend on your individual proportions.

✳ Place one long-folded blanket to support your torso.

✳ Place one square-folded blanket to support your head. Keep the loose end of the blanket toward your body so that the blanket can be tucked in to support your neck.

✳ Place one blanket to support each arm and your wrists.

✳ Recline on the blankets. You may cover your body with an additional blanket if you like.

✳ Rest, let go, recharge. It's a great idea to stay in this pose for as long as you can!

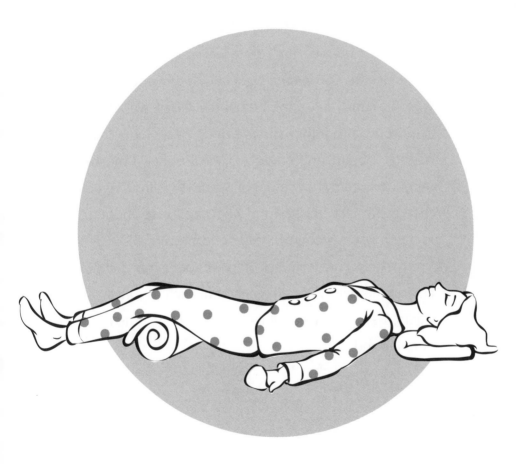

2

yogavitaminc

SNIFFLES, ALLERGIES, SORE throats, sluggishness— sometimes we don't quite feel sick, but we don't quite feel well either. So we reach for cough drops, keep Kleenex close at hand, and drink herbal tea. Often we ignore our symptoms altogether, but we don't necessarily feel fully healthy, vibrant, and energized. We wonder if maybe our immune system is low, but then we ask ourselves what does that really mean anyway, and what can we do about it? The immune system fights off viruses and infections; it's our built-in force field. But stress, lack of sleep, poor eating habits, and environmental toxins are constantly wearing away at the shield, leaving us vulnerable targets for any little bug that goes around.

YogaVitaminC can help bring our immune system back into balance. On a physical level, deep breathing will clear stale, stagnant air from the lungs, thus increasing respiration and circulation. Calming and steadying the nervous system will also strengthen the immune system. On a psychological and emotional level, practicing gentle, nurturing postures will increase our overall sense of well-being and awaken us to the importance of developing greater levels of self-care.

The sequence of YogaVitaminC poses in this chapter will bring your mind and body into equilibrium, giving your immune system just the jump-start it needs. Practice these postures with care, be gentle and loving with yourself, acknowledge your mind and body as precious gifts, and soon you'll feel it ... health!

* **heart-opening stretch**

* **posture-perfecting back bend**

* **propped-up angle pose**

* **reclining hero pose**

* **assisted forward bend**

* **chair back bend**

* **wall shoulder stand**

* **wide-legged plow pose**

* **simple legs-up-the-wall pose**

* **supported resting pose**

heart-opening stretch

HEART-OPENING STRETCH will gently release your thoracic spine and stretch your shoulders creating space across your chest.

you will need: *1 rolled mat or thin-rolled blanket*

✳ Place a rolled mat or thin-rolled blanket to support your shoulder blades.

✳ Recline on the prop, positioning the roll just beneath the shoulder blades across the upper back.

✳ Bend your arms to right angles, placing the backs of your hands on the floor.

✳ If your lower back is uncomfortable, bend your knees, placing your feet on the floor, wider than hip-distance apart, and allow your knees to come together for support.

✳ Close your eyes, breathe, and relax into the stretch for 3 minutes.

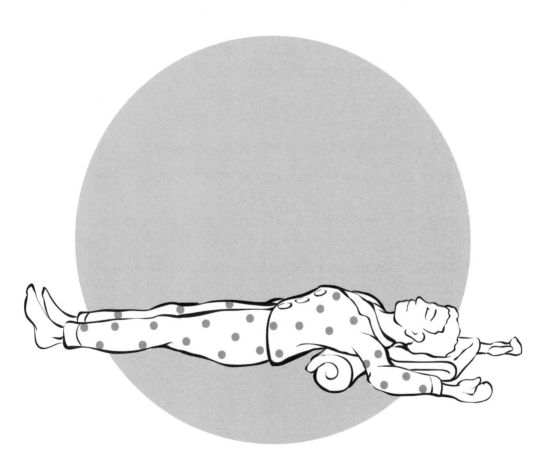

posture-perfecting back bend

POSTURE-PERFECTING BACK BEND stimulates the thymus gland, shoring up your body's internal defense.

you will need: *2 blocks*

* Place two blocks to support your head and shoulder blades.

* Recline on the blocks. Allow your arms to rest at your sides, palms facing the ceiling.

* Either stretch your legs straight, or bend your knees, placing your feet wider than hip-distance apart and allowing the knees to rest together for support.

* Close your eyes, breathe, and surrender onto the blocks for 3 minutes.

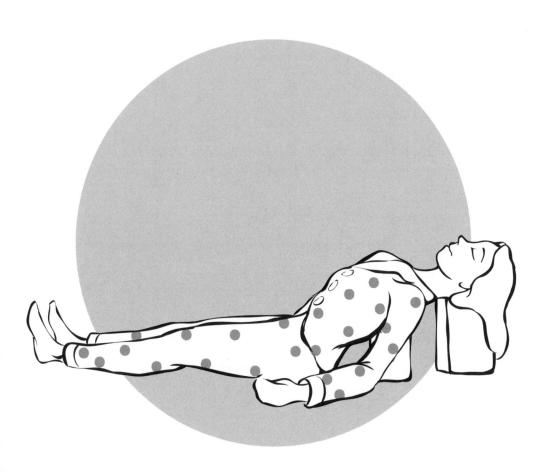

propped-up angle pose

PROPPED-UP ANGLE Pose creates perfect spinal alignment, allowing long, smooth breathing.

you will need: *a wall, 2 blocks*

* Sitting with your back against a wall for support, bring the soles of your feet together, heels 3 to 12 inches from you, depending on what you find comfortable.

* Place a block under each knee for support.

* Place your hands comfortably in your lap, one on each knee, either palms up or down.

* Gently press the outer feet into each other, promoting a gentle inner thigh and hip stretch.

* Lift from the base of the spine through the crown of the head.

* Close your eyes, breathe, and hold for 2 to 5 minutes.

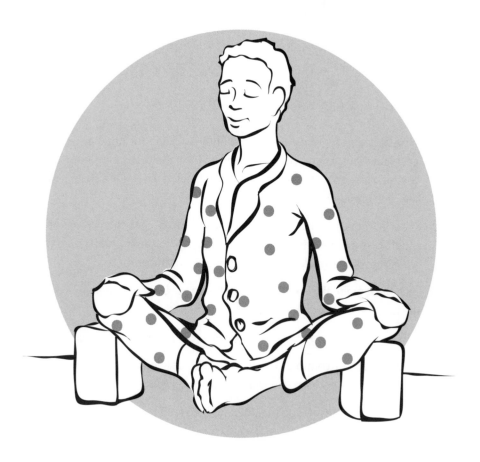

reclining hero pose

RECLINING HERO POSE opens the chest while providing a gentle stretch for the hip flexors.

you will need: *4 blankets and/or 2 bolsters*

✳ Place bolsters and/or blankets in a slightly modified T-formation. Use at least four blankets and/or two bolsters to form the base of the T, and stagger the blankets/bolsters to create a slight incline. From the side, the blankets will resemble a set of stairs.

✳ Kneel in front of the bolsters/blankets with your back to them. Your knees should be together, with your feet, soles facing up, slightly wider than your hips. Rest your buttocks on the bottom "stair" of the props.

✳ Lean back, gradually lowering yourself onto the bolsters/blankets. If this seems impossible, add more blankets to the base of the T.

✳ Rest your arms alongside your body, with your palms facing the ceiling.

✳ If you feel any discomfort in your lower back, use your hands to ease your buttock flesh away from you while lengthening your lower back.

✳ Close your eyes, let go and breathe, and hold for 3 to 10 minutes.

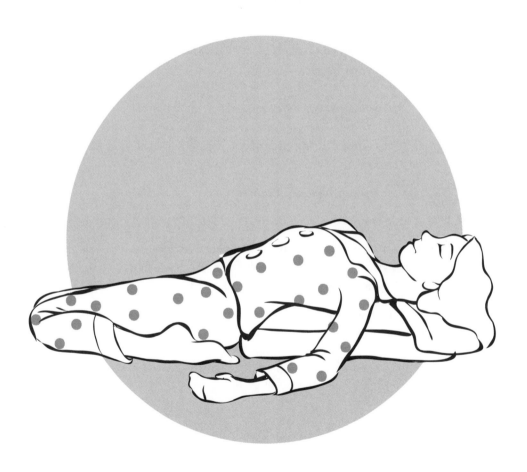

assisted forward bend

ASSISTED FORWARD BEND will release tightness from your lower back and tension from your neck.

you will need: *1 square-folded blanket, 1 block, 1 strap*

✳ Sit with your sit bones on the edge of one square-folded blanket. Keep your legs outstretched.

✳ Place a block against the soles of your feet.

✳ Loop a strap around the block, holding one side of the strap in each hand.

✳ Keeping your chest lifted and the back of your neck long, start to walk your hands down the strap to gently stretch the backs of your legs (keeping your knees slightly bent if you find it more comfortable).

✳ Use your shoulders to pull down your back and keep your chest open. Hold for 1 to 3 minutes.

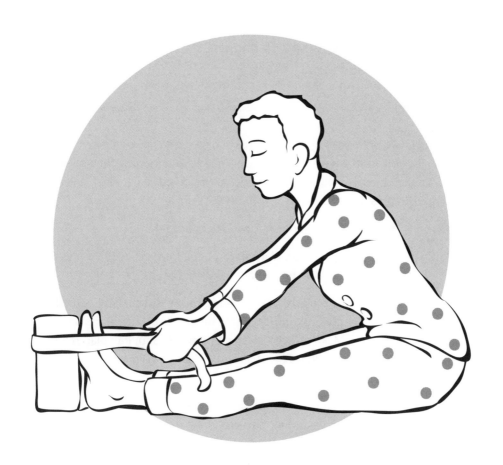

chair back bend

CHAIR BACK BEND is very stimulating, as it increases blood flow to the head, arms, and legs.

you will need: *a sturdy chair, 2 or 3 long-folded blankets, 1 stool or high stack of blankets, 1 nonslip mat*

* Place two or three long-folded blankets, depending on your height (the taller you are, the fewer blankets you'll need), with the short end of the blankets between the legs of a sturdy, open-backed chair—the blankets extending at least 18 inches away from the front legs of the chair.

* Place a nonslip mat on the chair for skid resistance.

* Place a stool or high stack of blankets/bolsters, the same height as the seat of the chair, one leg's distance from the back of the chair.

* Sit backward on the chair, straddling it, and gently ease your hips forward, holding on to the chair for support, until your middle back is resting on the seat of the chair. Make sure the bottom tips of your shoulder blades are resting on the front edge of the chair and the crown of your head is resting on the blankets.

* Place your feet through the back of the chair and onto the stool/blankets, and thread your hands through the legs of the chair, holding on to the back of the legs for stability.

✳ Close your eyes, let go and breathe, and hold for 30 seconds to 3 minutes.

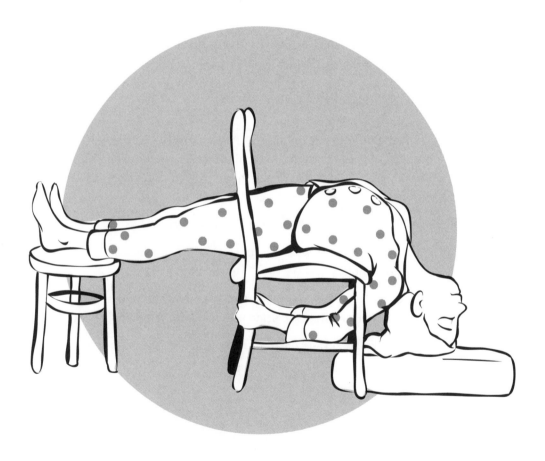

wall shoulder stand

WALL SHOULDER STAND activates the glands located in the neck, including the thyroid, restoring their proper functioning.

you will need: *a wall, 2 open-folded blankets*

✳ Begin in the Simple Legs-Up-the-Wall Pose (see pg. 48), with your torso and shoulders supported by two open-folded blankets and your head and neck off the blankets. Be sure to have the smooth folded edges facing toward your neck.

✳ Bend your knees and place your feet flat on the wall.

✳ Gently press against the wall with your feet, lifting your hips until your body forms a right angle.

✳ Interlace your hands behind you, and roll your shoulders underneath you for support. You may also try placing your hands on your middle back.

✳ Close your eyes, let go and breathe, and hold for 3 to 10 minutes.

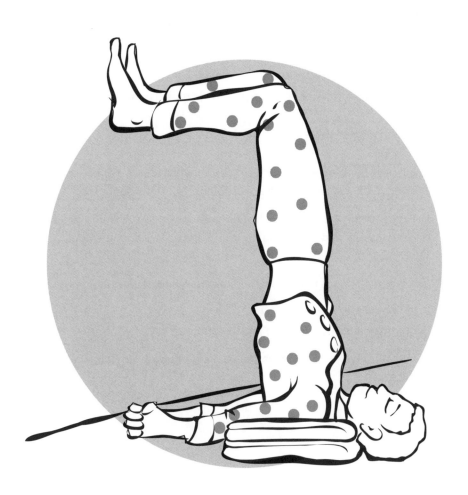

wide-legged plow pose

WIDE-LEGGED PLOW releases the lower back after Wall Shoulder Stand and also encourages the proper functioning of the lymph system.

you will need: *2 open-folded blankets*

✳ Begin by lying down with your torso and shoulders on two open-folded blankets, with the smooth edge of the blankets facing your head.

✳ With your palms pressing into the floor for support, swing your legs up and back over your head, lifting your hips, until the balls of your feet touch the floor.

✳ Interlace your hands behind you and roll your shoulders underneath you.

✳ Walk your feet away from each other until your legs form a wide V-shape. Bend your knees slightly if that's more comfortable.

✳ Close your eyes, let go and breathe, and hold this pose for 30 seconds to 3 minutes.

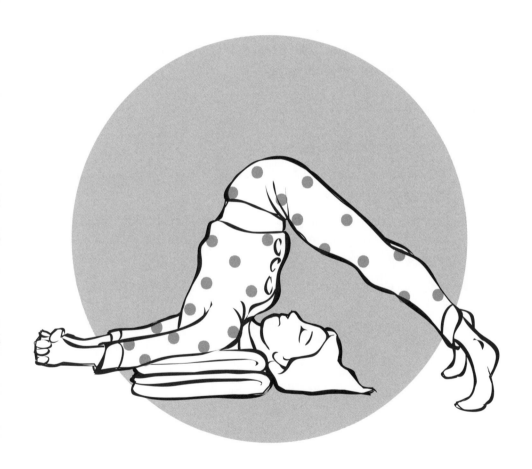

simple legs-up-the-wall pose

SIMPLE LEGS-UP-THE-WALL POSE brings blood and lymph fluid into the belly, recharging the internal organs.

you will need: *a wall*

* Sit with your right side to the wall.

* Support yourself with your left hand as you swing your legs up the wall and recline on your back.

* Place your hands over your shoulders and turn your palms to the floor. Push yourself toward the wall so that your hips are as close to it as is comfortably possible.

* Close your eyes, let go and breathe, and hold for 3 to 5 minutes.

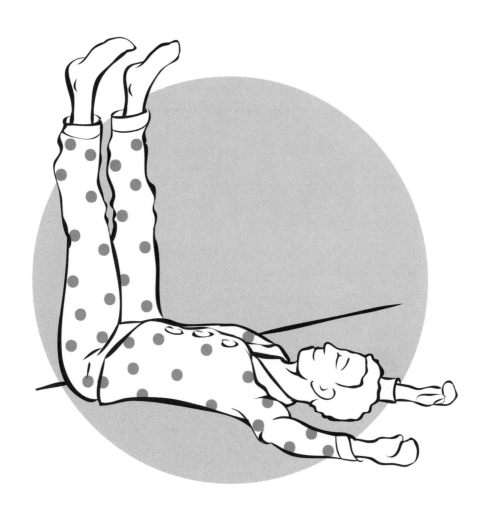

supported resting pose

SUPPORTED RESTING POSE allows the mind and body to completely relax and gain strength to face any immunity attack.

you will need: *1 square-folded blanket, 1 thick-rolled blanket*

✳ Place a square-folded blanket to support your head and a thick-rolled blanket to support your knees. The exact placement of the blankets will depend on your particular proportions.

✳ Recline on the blankets, resting your arms alongside your body with your palms facing the ceiling.

✳ Close your eyes, let go, and breathe for 3 to 10 minutes.

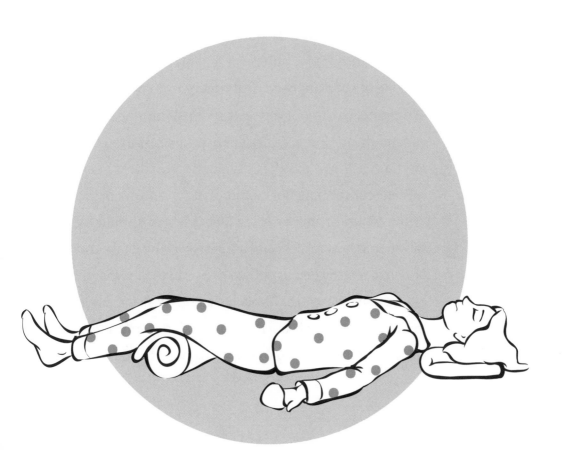

3

yogaalarmclock

NODDING OFF BY noontime? Dragging your feet far before Friday? If you're feeling heavy and slow or backing out of plans because the less you do, the less you feel like doing, you're not alone. It seems that many of us are constantly tired, unable to get our engines started or break inertia's spell. We have the attention span of three-year-olds, we can't concentrate, our memory is fuzzy, and our moods are at the whim of the weather. Sleep, which should be our salvation, is now restless and unsatisfying. And it takes our last ounce of energy just to get out of bed in the morning. How did we end up like this? It's likely that physical and emotional tension has built up in our muscles, making them knotted and stiff, and in turn making us sluggish and sedentary.

Fortunately, the YogaAlarmClock poses in this chapter can help us to wake up our muscles and our minds. Unlike most styles of exercise, restorative yoga doesn't expend energy, it actually puts energy back! Many of the poses here focus on improving posture—the more upright we hold our bodies, the more awake and alert we feel.

Just as inertia can perpetuate sleepiness, once we get going, inertia kicks in to keep us moving. So if we can stop listing reasons not to act, tell our chattering brains to butt out, and get into our first pose, our newfound energy will be all the motivation we need to continue. And not long from now, when that alarm clock buzzes in the morning, lo and behold, we'll feel … awake!

* **hero on a throne pose**

* **strap shoulder stretch**

* **supported boat pose**

* **chair back bend at the wall**

* **wall-walking back bend**

* **climbing locust**

* **wall knee hug**

* **straight-leg wall twist**

* **legs-up-the-wall with props**

hero on a throne pose

HERO ON A THRONE POSE relieves stiff hips, knees, and ankles as it coaxes the mind and sharpens the senses.

you will need: *1 block*

✳ From a kneeling position, place a block between your feet, the narrow ends of the block touching the inner edges of your feet.

✳ Bring your inner knees together and sit down on the block. Adjust the height of the block according to your flexibility, and use an additional block if necessary.

✳ Place your palms facedown on your thighs, draw your shoulder blades down your back, and lengthen your spine from its base through the crown of your head.

✳ If you feel any tenderness in your knees, use more blocks.

✳ Extend through your big toes and draw your outer ankles in.

✳ Close your eyes, let go and breathe, and hold for 1 to 5 minutes.

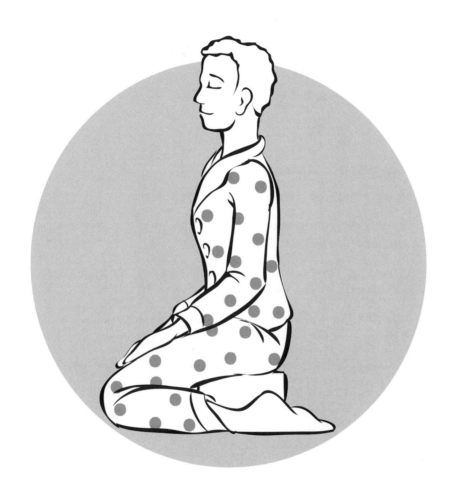

strap shoulder stretch

STRAP SHOULDER STRETCH opens the shoulders, one of the key components of healthy posture.

you will need: *1 block, 1 strap*

* Begin in Hero on a Throne Pose (see pg. 54).

* Place one end of an unlooped strap in each hand.

* Straighten your arms in front of you, and slide your hands away from each other until they are between $2^1/_2$ and 3 feet apart.

* Keeping your arms straight, and your hands gripping the strap, lift your arms up and over your head.

* Adjust the distance between your hands so that you can keep your arms straight yet still feel a significant stretch in your shoulders.

* Close your eyes, let go and breathe, and hold. Repeat in fluid movements 10 to 15 times.

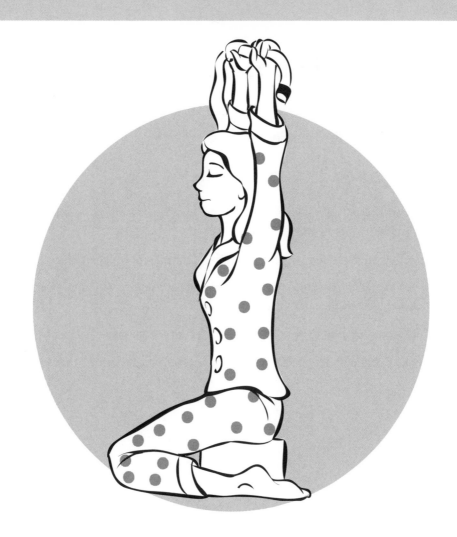

supported boat pose

SUPPORTED BOAT POSE is an active pose that increases circulation and strengthens the muscles in the back and legs.

you will need: *1 strap*

* Sit with your knees bent and the soles of your feet flat on the floor, heels roughly 12 inches from your buttocks.

* Loop a strap around your upper back and the balls of your feet.

* Keeping your chest lifted, carefully lean back, lifting your feet until your lower legs are parallel to the floor.

* Extend your arms in front of you, palms facing each other.

* Close your eyes, let go and breathe, and hold this position for 30 seconds.

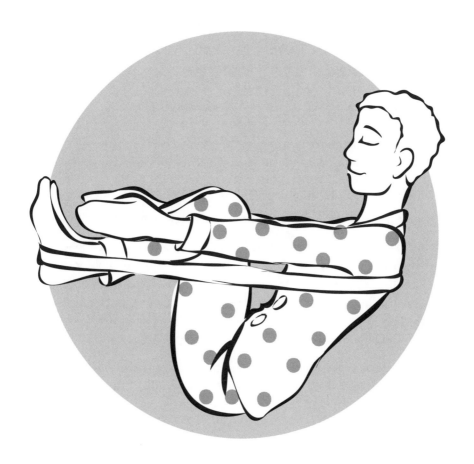

chair back bend at the wall

CHAIR BACK BEND AT THE WALL is extremely invigorating, increasing flexibility in the spine and building stamina.

you will need: *a wall, a sturdy chair, 2 or 3 long-folded blankets, 1 nonslip mat*

* Place the short end of two or three long-folded blankets between the legs of a sturdy chair (adjust the number of blankets according to your height).

* Place a nonslip mat on the chair for skid resistance.

* Place the back of the chair 2 feet from a wall, preferably on a smooth surface.

* Sit backward on the chair, straddling it. Press your feet against the wall, where the wall meets the floor, and then gently ease your hips forward and slide the chair away from the wall. Hold on to the chair for support, easing your hips forward until your middle back is resting on the chair. Make sure the bottom tips of your shoulder blades are resting on the front edge of the chair and the crown of your head is resting on the blankets.

* If you are on a carpet, manually adjust the distance between the chair and the wall so that when you are in the full pose, your feet can press against the wall for support.

✳ Close your eyes, let go and breathe, and hold for 30 seconds to 3 minutes.

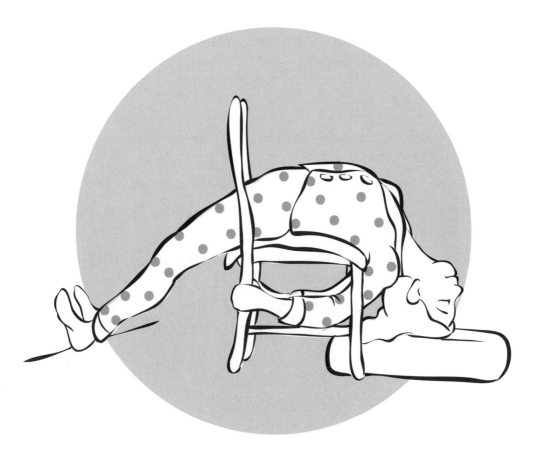

wall-walking back bend

WALL-WALKING BACK BEND challenges your mind and your body, creating a sense of accomplishment.

you will need: *a wall*

✳ Stand about 2 feet from the wall, with your feet parallel to each other and hip-distance apart.

✳ Bring your hands together in a prayer position in front of your heart.

✳ Begin to lean back, lifting your chest and taking the prayer position up and over your head until your hands touch the wall.

✳ Relax, breathe, and if your flexibility warrants, separate your hands shoulder distance and start to walk them down the wall.

✳ Reverse your movements, walking your hands up the wall and ending where you began, standing with your hands in front of your heart in prayer position.

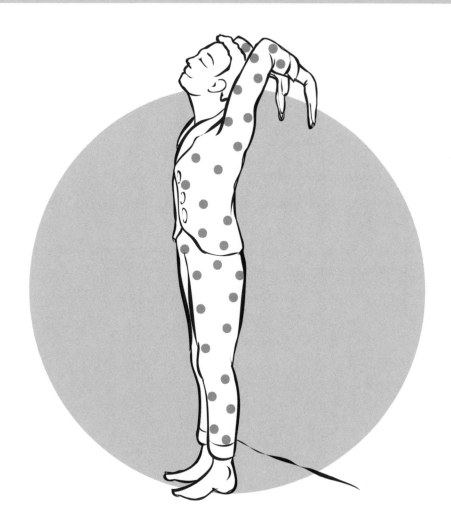

YOGA ALARM CLOCK

climbing locust

CLIMBING LOCUST eases into the shoulders and the upper back.

you will need: *a wall*

* Lie facedown with your head 1 to 2 feet from the wall.

* Begin walking your hands up the wall, focusing on bringing your upper back into an arch.

* Walk your hands up the wall until your arms are straight and you feel a sensation of hanging from the wall.

* Close your eyes, let go and breathe, and hold for 30 seconds to 3 minutes.

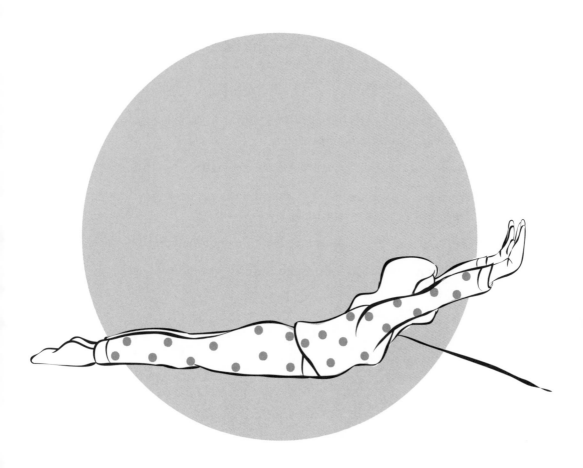

YOGAALARMCLOCK

wall knee hug

WALL KNEE HUG releases the spine after back-bending work.

you will need: *a wall, 1 strap*

* ✳ Begin in the Simple Legs-Up-the-Wall Pose (see pg. 48), with your ankles secured together using a strap.

* ✳ Bend your knees, sliding your heels down the wall.

* ✳ Keep your hips on the floor and allow your knees to move toward your armpits until your feet are flat against the wall.

* ✳ Rest your arms alongside your body with your palms facing the ceiling.

* ✳ Close your eyes, let go and breathe, and hold for 2 to 5 minutes.

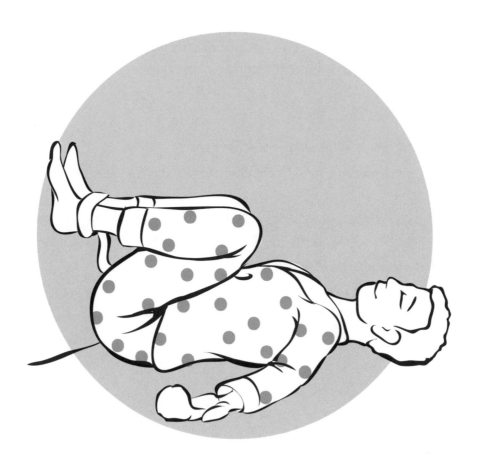

straight-leg wall twist

STRAIGHT-LEG WALL TWIST continues to release the back while yawning open the sides of the body.

you will need: *a wall*

* Begin in the Simple Legs-Up-the-Wall Pose (see pg. 48).

* Stretch your arms to your sides, palms down, forming a T-shape with your body.

* Take a deep breath in, and as you exhale, lower your legs to the right. Keep your knees slightly bent if that's more comfortable for you.

* Turn your chin toward your left shoulder.

* Close your eyes, let go and breathe, and hold for 1 to 3 minutes. Repeat with legs going to the left side and chin toward the right.

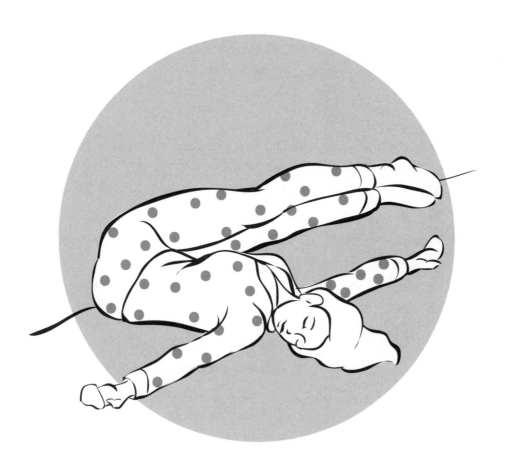

YOGA ALARM CLOCK

legs-up-the-wall with props

LEGS-UP-THE-WALL WITH PROPS allows the mind and body to settle and integrate a newfound sense of vitality.

you will need: *a wall, 2 to 4 long-folded blankets or 1 to 2 bolsters, 1 strap*

✳ Stack two to four long-folded blankets, or one to two bolsters, and place them 4 to 6 inches from the wall, running parallel to it.

✳ Sit sideways on the middle of the blankets/bolster(s), with your right side to the wall.

✳ Support yourself with your left hand as you swing your legs up the wall and recline on your back.

✳ Reverse your hands by your shoulders, placing your palms flat with your fingertips pointing toward your shoulders, and pressing into the floor for leverage, adjust yourself so that your lower back is on the blankets/bolster, and your sit bones are resting in the space between the props and the wall.

✳ Once situated, bend your knees and tighten a strap around your shins.

✳ Extend your legs back up the wall (keep your knees slightly bent if that's more comfortable for you). Make sure the strap is tight enough so that keeping your legs extended is effortless.

➡

✳ Close your eyes, let go and breathe, and hold for 3 to 8 minutes.

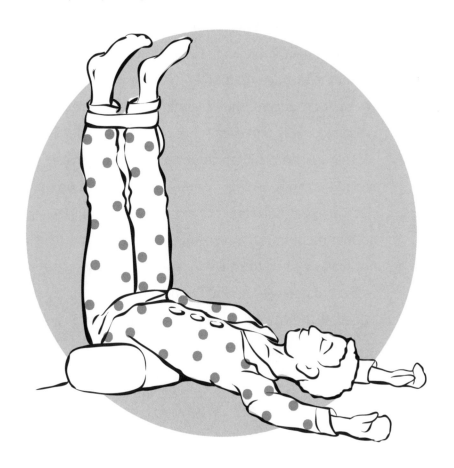

4

yogalullaby

WE'VE ALL BEEN there—mind racing, eyes wide, staring at the ceiling at 3 AM. We toss, turn, count sheep; we may even pace, read, or reorganize our closets. But what we can't do, despite the valiant efforts of eye masks, white noise machines, and memory foam pillows, is sleep. Insomnia may be chronic, intermittent, or rare, but even one sleepless night can have significant negative effects on us. With our fast-paced lives and many responsibilities—jobs, appointments, and family—not to mention interests and hobbies, we need to be awake and alert. We bring our daily worries to bed with us and flounder for tools to help us fall asleep, all the while growing increasingly tense as we anticipate our groggy, puffy-eyed morning.

When we were children, our parents held and sang to us till we drifted off to dreamland. YogaLullaby can help rock us into a deep, restful, long night's sleep. Restorative yoga postures still our central nervous system, slow our breathing, and, with practice, help free us from incessant mental laundry lists. A good night's sleep comes when we are actually tired, relaxed, safe, and supported, and our bodies are warm and comfortable, our brains noise-free.

The sequence of YogaLullaby poses in this chapter will calm and quiet the mind while soothing and relaxing the body. In each posture, focus on lengthening your breath, especially when you exhale. Let yourself slow down, and before you know it … *zzzzzzzzzzzz!*

✳ **leaning forward bend**

✳ **resting dog pose**

✳ **lounging hero pose**

✳ **relaxing forward bend**

✳ **supported bound angle pose**

✳ **assisted shoulder stand**

✳ **effortless plow pose**

✳ **simple supported back bend**

✳ **grounding resting pose**

leaning forward bend

LEANING FORWARD BEND gently stretches the backs of the legs while encouraging the shoulders, neck, and facial muscles to relax.

you will need: *a wall*

* Stand with your back to the wall, about a foot away from it, with your feet hip-distance apart and parallel.

* Keep your feet planted and lean back until your hips rest on the wall. You may keep your knees slightly bent if that's more comfortable.

* Fold forward, allowing your torso, neck, and head to relax completely.

* Hold your elbows with opposite hands, close your eyes, let go and breathe, and hold for 1 to 4 minutes.

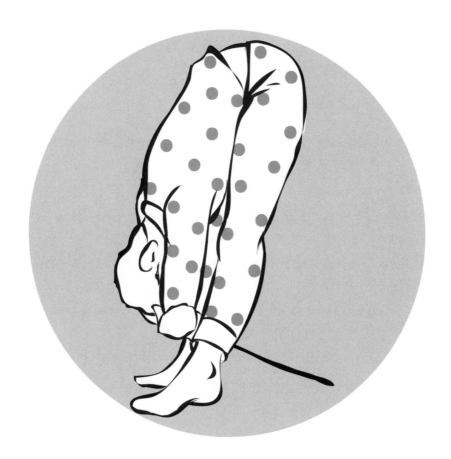

resting dog pose

RESTING DOG POSE supports the head to calm the mind while allowing the backs of the legs to yawn open.

you will need: *1 block*

* Kneel on all fours, with your knees directly underneath your hips, and your hands, knees, and feet hip-distance apart.

* Place a block on the floor below your chest.

* Make sure the creases in your wrists run directly perpendicular to your torso and that your arms are perfectly straight.

* Curl your toes under, press into your flat palms, and lift your knees up and away from the floor.

* Keeping your knees slightly bent, press into your hands until you form a straight line from your hands to your hips.

* Rest your head on the block, adjusting its height as necessary.

* Try to straighten your legs to increase the stretch if doing so is comfortable for you.

✳ Close your eyes, let go and breathe, and hold for 30 seconds to 2 minutes.

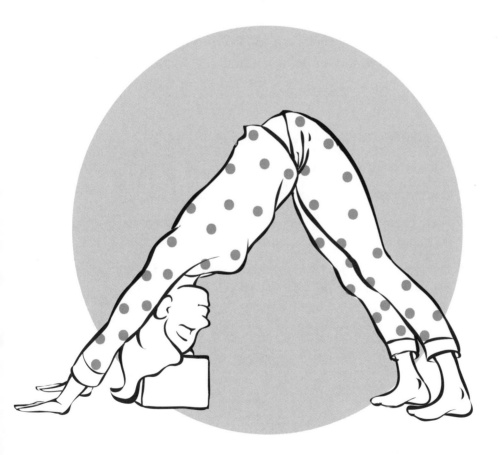

lounging hero pose

LOUNGING HERO POSE melts tension from your lower back and hips while continuing to settle mental chatter.

you will need: *2 blocks*

    ✳ Begin in the Hero on a Throne Pose (see pg. 54)

    ✳ Place an additional block on its end in front of you for support.

    ✳ Fold forward, resting your forehead on the block.

    ✳ Find a comfortable position for your arms, either in front of you or alongside your body, with your palms facing the ceiling.

    ✳ Close your eyes, let go of your shoulders completely, and breathe into the backside of your body for 2 to 5 minutes.

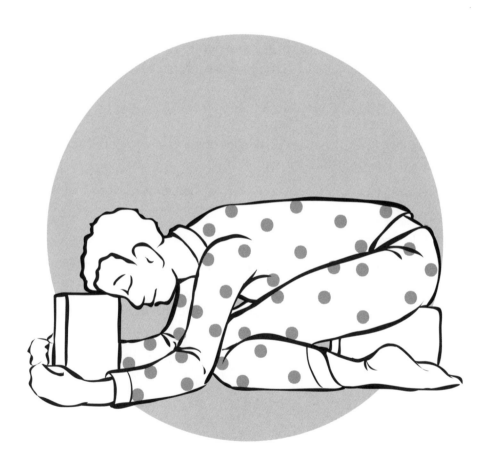

relaxing forward bend

RELAXING FORWARD BEND provides a gentle stretch for the back of the legs and hips while allowing the head and torso to rest completely.

you will need: *1 square-folded blanket, 1 to 4 long-folded blankets or bolsters*

* Sit with just your sit bones on the edge of one square-folded blanket, keeping your legs together and outstretched.

* Place one to four long-folded blankets or a bolster/blanket combination on top of your legs.

* Fold forward at your hips and rest your torso on the blankets.

* If you feel any discomfort in your knees, place a rolled blanket under them for support.

* Close your eyes, let go and breathe deeply, and hold for 1 to 5 minutes.

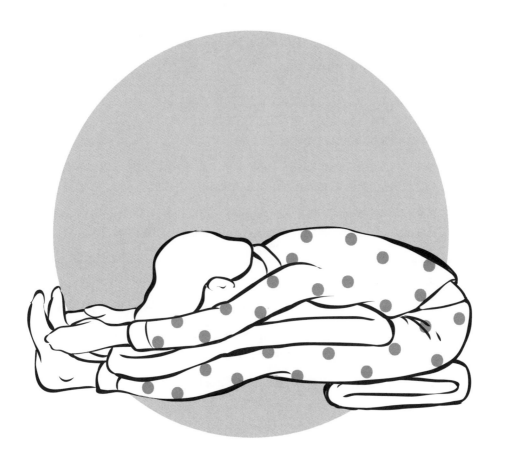

supported bound angle pose

SUPPORTED BOUND ANGLE POSE gently releases the inner thighs and passively opens the hips.

you will need: *1 to 3 long-folded blankets, 1 strap, 2 blocks (optional)*

* Place bolsters and/or blankets into a T-formation.

* Sit directly in front of the short end of the blankets/bolster, and bring the soles of your feet together with your heels 6 inches from you.

* Place a wide-looped strap over your shoulders, tightening it around your lower back and around the tops and outer edges of the feet.

* Recline on the blankets/bolsters, resting your arms alongside your body, palms facing the ceiling.

* If your knees are uncomfortable, place a block under each knee for support.

* If your lower back aches, use your hands to ease the flesh of your buttocks away from you, lengthening your lower back.

* Close your eyes, let go and breathe, and hold for 3 to 5 minutes.

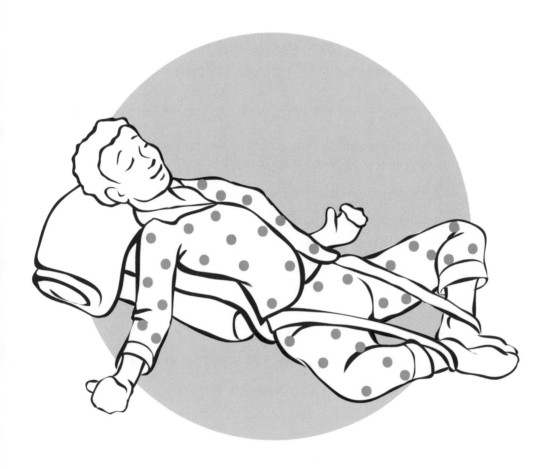

assisted shoulder stand

ASSISTED SHOULDER STAND stimulates the thyroid gland and improves circulation, creating a very relaxed, steady feeling in the body.

you will need: *1 bolster or 2 long-folded blankets, a sturdy chair, 1 nonslip mat or blanket*

＊ Place a bolster or two long-folded blankets with their smooth edge out directly in front of the legs of a sturdy chair.

＊ Cover the seat of the chair with a nonslip mat or a blanket.

＊ Sit sideways on the chair. Holding on to the sides of the the chair back, swing your legs over the top of the back.

＊ Slide your buttocks forward, and ease your shoulders down onto the bolster/blankets, resting your head on the floor.

＊ Thread your hands through the front legs of the chair, holding on to the back legs.

＊ Continuing to hold on to the chair, slowly straighten your legs, one at a time.

＊ Your lower back should rest comfortably on the edge of the chair.

＊ Reach up through the balls of your feet.

✳ Close your eyes, let go and breathe, and hold for 3 to 5 minutes.

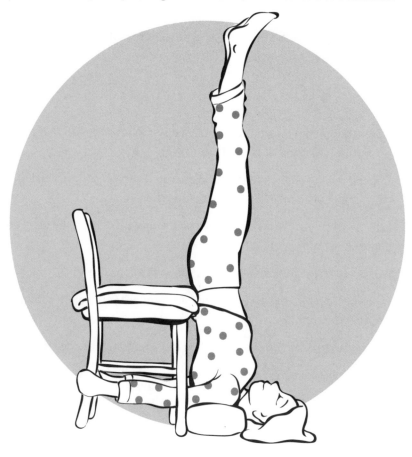

YOGALULLABY

effortless plow pose

EFFORTLESS PLOW POSE allows for greater circulation throughout the body, encouraging relaxation.

you will need: *1 bolster or 2 long-folded blankets—more as needed, a sturdy chair*

* Place a bolster or two long-folded blankets, smooth edges out, 6 inches from the back legs of a sturdy chair.

* Depending on your height (the taller you are, the more lift you'll need), stack any number of blankets on the seat of the chair.

* Lie down with your head facing the chair, your shoulders on the blankets, and your head and neck off the blankets.

* Bend your knees and place your feet flat on the floor.

* Push your feet into the floor, lift your hips, interlock your hands behind you, and roll your shoulders underneath you.

* Swing your legs up and overhead, then rest your thighs on the chair.

* Release your hands, resting your arms by your head, palms facing the ceiling.

* Close your eyes, let go onto the support of the props and breathe, holding your position for 3 minutes.

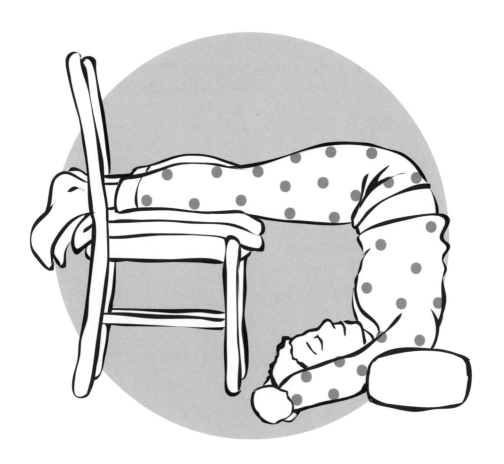

simple supported back bend

SIMPLE SUPPORTED BACK BEND completely supports the neck in a vulnerable, heart-opening pose, allowing the mind to become accustomed to the vulnerability sometimes associated with deep sleep.

you will need: *1 thick-rolled blanket, 1 thin-rolled blanket*

✳ Place a thick-rolled blanket where it will support your middle back.

✳ Place a thin-rolled blanket where it will support your neck.

✳ Recline on the blankets.

✳ Position your feet a little wider than hip-distance apart and your arms palms-up 6 to 12 inches from your body.

✳ Close your eyes, let go and breathe, and hold for 3 to 8 minutes.

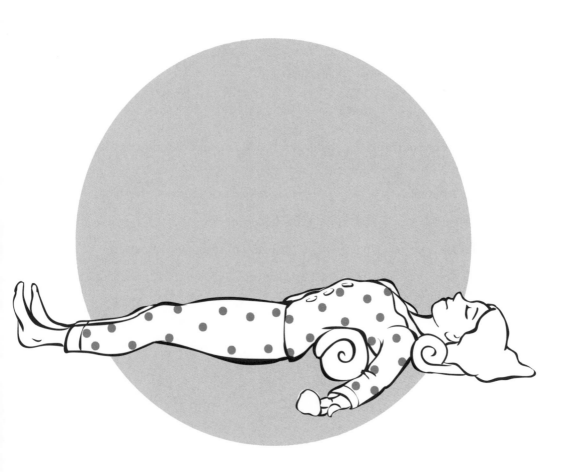

grounding resting pose

GROUNDING RESTING POSE uses the weight of blankets to encourage the body to drop and let go fully.

you will need: *1 partially rolled square-folded blanket, 1 bolster or 2 to 3 long-folded blankets*

✳ Lie on your back. Place partially rolled square-folded blanket under your neck and head for support.

✳ Place a bolster or two to three long-folded blankets over your thighs.

✳ Extend your arms alongside your body, with your palms facing the ceiling.

✳ Allow the weight of the bolster/blankets to encourage you to let go.

✳ Close your eyes, let go and breathe deeply, holding your position for 5 to 10 minutes.

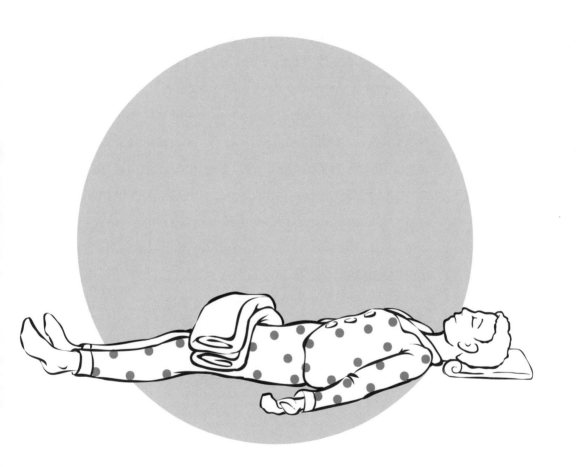

yogabackrub

WHATEVER THE CAUSE, we can't escape the truth: our backs sometimes hurt—they ache, they pinch, they seize up. From our neck and shoulders, all the way down our spines, our muscles become sore and stiff and our bones feel totally out of joint. There are so many reasons why we may suffer: we sit too long, we have poor posture, our stomach and back muscles are weak. And let's face it, the more stressed and worried we get, the more we tense and squeeze our poor overtaxed, undercared-for muscles, which only makes our back problems worse.

What we really need is a nice, soothing YogaBackRub. Perhaps the greatest gift we can give our struggling back muscles is time and space to relax. Easing muscular tension will put less pressure on the vertebrae and encourage proper spinal alignment. The sequence of YogaBackRub poses in this chapter will stretch and strengthen your back, providing both long- and short-term relief for back pain.

The first three poses gently warm up your body and ease tension. But the last five poses in the sequence are the real miracle workers, focusing on increasing hip flexibility to alleviate any locked or frozen sensations in your lower back, as well as stretching the leg muscles to improve mobility.

As always, take your time with these postures, and never do any pose that intensifies your pain. Be patient with your back; allow it to rest, heal, and get stronger gradually. Allow yourself to respect the process of healing and you'll be greatly rewarded.

* **stretching dog pose**

* **lifted camel pose**

* **wall twist**

* **reclining big toe posture**

* **twisting reclining big toe posture**

* **reclining wide-leg pose**

* **bound angle at the wall**

* **pigeon at the wall**

* **lower back reset**

* **knee hug with strap**

stretching dog pose

STRETCHING DOG POSE gently warms the body, opening the shoulders and the backs of the legs. Working with the block in this pose actually helps the lower back broaden and release.

you will need: *a wall, 1 block*

* Kneel on all fours facing a wall, with your knees directly underneath your hips.

* Place a block, positioned at its narrowest width, between your legs.

* Place your thumb and index finger against the wall, palms flat to the floor and shoulder-distance apart.

* Curl your toes under, press into your palms, and slowly lift your knees up and away from the floor until your body forms a straight line from your wrists to your hips.

* Relax your head and neck and firm your thighs, gradually straightening your legs.

* Once in the posture, inwardly roll your inner thighs as though you were attempting to shoot the block away from you.

* Continue to press into your hands, lengthening your spine.

✳ Close your eyes, let go and breathe, and hold for 30 seconds to 2 minutes.

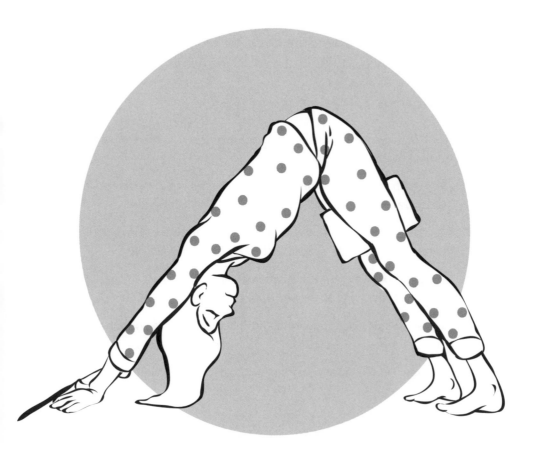

YOGABACKRUB

lifted camel pose

LIFTED CAMEL POSE opens the chest, tackling the all-too-common, pain-causing slouch.

you will need: *a low table, 2 bolsters or 4 long-folded blankets*

✳ Use a low table, 14 to 24 inches high (or you may use a higher table and lift the floor by placing blankets beside it).

✳ Place two bolsters or four long-folded blankets on top of the table, with at least two additional blankets on top of the far blanket/bolster.

✳ Kneel on the floor facing away from the table, with your calves underneath the table. The top of the props should be just below your waist.

✳ Gently lean back, reclining on your forearms. Lift your chest and relax the backside of your body on the props.

✳ Make sure your neck is supported, and find a comfortable position for your arms.

✳ Close your eyes, let go and breathe, and hold for 1 to 3 minutes.

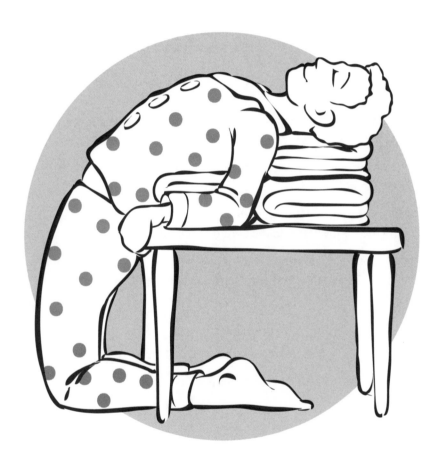

YOGABACKRUB

wall twist

WALL TWIST elongates the spinal muscles, relieving tension.

you will need: *a wall and blanket or bolster (optional)*

✳ Sit with your back 6 inches away from a wall in a comfortable cross-legged position, elevating your hips with a blanket or bolster if necessary.

✳ From your waist, turn to the right, placing your left hand on your right knee and your right hand on the wall.

✳ Lift your chest, pull your shoulders down your back, and using the wall for leverage, gently ease into the twist on each exhale.

✳ Close your eyes, let go and breathe, and hold the twist for 30 seconds to 2 minutes. Return to center, and then repeat on the other side.

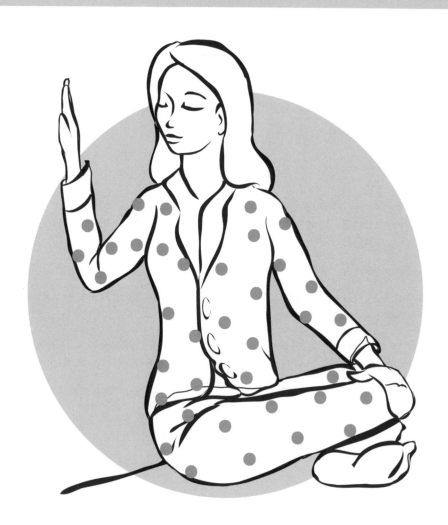

YOGABACKRUB

reclining big toe posture

RECLINING BIG TOE POSTURE will spread the lower back and relieve pain in the sacrum.

you will need: *a wall, 1 strap, 1 block*

❋ Lie down on your back with your feet together and pressing against a wall. Place a block about 2 feet from the wall and one leg's distance from the right side of your body.

❋ Draw your right knee into your chest.

❋ Loop a strap around the ball of your right foot and slowly ease your leg out until it is straight.

❋ Place both ends of the strap into your right hand. Pressing the left foot against the wall, slowly lower your leg to the right until it rests on a block.

❋ Extend your left arm away from you, palm facing the ceiling, and turn your chin toward your left shoulder.

❋ Close your eyes, let go and breathe, and hold the pose for up to 2 minutes.

❋ Reverse the motion, return to the beginning, and repeat on the other side.

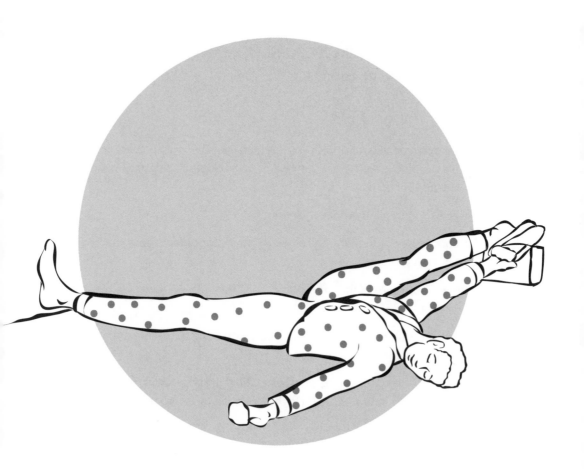

twisting reclining big toe posture

TWISTING RECLINING BIG TOE POSTURE will open the lower back while gently stretching the outer hips.

you will need: *a wall, 1 strap, 1 block*

* Lie down on your back with your feet together and pressing against a wall. Place a block about 2 feet from the wall and one leg's distance from the left side of your body.

* Draw your right knee into your chest.

* Loop a strap around the ball of your right foot and slowly ease your leg out until it is straight.

* Place both ends of the strap into your left hand. Slowly lower your leg to the left until it rests on a block.

* Extend your right arm away from you, palm facing the ceiling, and turn your chin toward your right shoulder.

* Close your eyes, let go and breathe, and hold the pose for up to 2 minutes. Reverse the motion, returning to the beginning, and repeat on the other side.

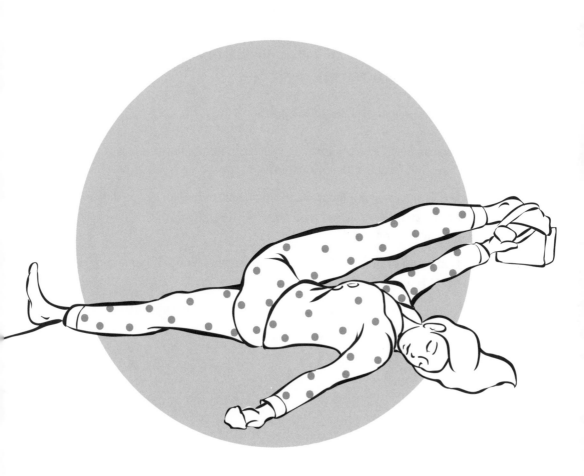

reclining wide-leg pose

RECLINING WIDE-LEG POSE will gently stretch your inner thighs relieving tension in the hips and lower back.

you will need: *a wall, 1 thin-folded blanket (optional)*

* Begin in the Simple Legs-Up-the-Wall Pose (see pg. 48), with or without a thin-folded blanket under your hips.

* Flex your feet, extending through your heels. Allow your legs to slide away from each other until they form a wide V-shape. Keep your legs bent slightly if it's more comfortable.

* Find a comfortable position for your arms, either alongside your body or next to your head, palms facing the ceiling.

* Close your eyes, let go and breathe, and hold for 1 to 3 minutes.

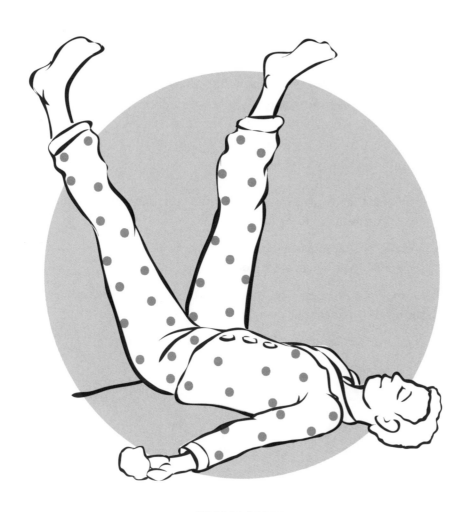

YOGABACKRUB

bound angle at the wall

BOUND ANGLE AT WALL POSE provides an excellent opportunity for slow breathing and meditation while gently lengthening the inner thighs.

you will need: *a wall, 1 thin-folded blanket (optional)*

✳ Begin in the Simple Legs-Up-the-Wall Pose (see pg. 48), with or without a thin-folded blanket under your hips.

✳ Bring the soles of your feet together and allow your heels to slide toward you, bending your knees to the sides.

✳ Once in the posture, press the outer edges of your feet toward each other, and gently lengthen your inner thighs.

✳ Close your eyes, let go and breathe, and hold for 1 to 3 minutes.

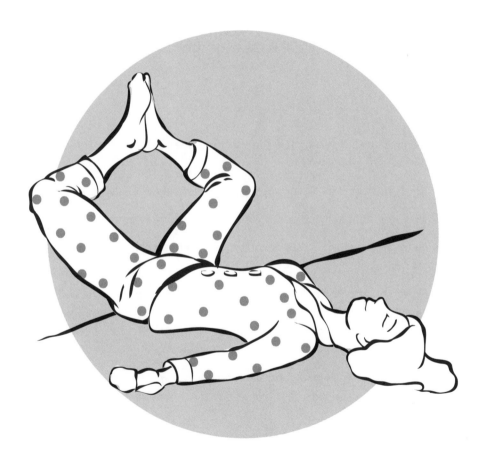

YOGABACKRUB

pigeon at the wall

PIGEON AT THE WALL POSE is ideal for stretching and opening your outer thighs.

you will need: *a wall, 1 thin-folded blanket (optional)*

* Begin in the Simple Legs-Up-the-Wall Pose (see pg. 48), with or without a low blanket under your hips.

* Cross your right ankle over your left thigh just below your left knee.

* Flex your right foot and gently ease your right knee away from you.

* Begin sliding your left foot down the wall, stopping before your hips lift off the floor.

* As you breathe and hold, consider sliding your left heel down the wall until your left foot is flat on the wall with the leg bent to a 90 degree angle, but not at the expense of lifting your hips or allowing them to slide away from the wall.

* Close your eyes, let go and breathe, and hold for 1 to 3 minutes. Then slide your legs back up the wall and repeat on the other side.

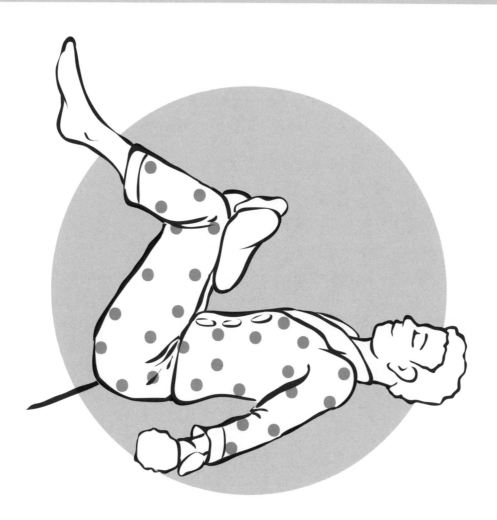

YOGABACKRUB

lower back reset

LOWER BACK RESET realigns the pelvis, which, due to poor posture and tight leg muscles, tends to "tilt" forward, putting pressure on the lower back.

you will need: *nothing*

※ Lie on your back, hugging your knees into your chest.

※ Interlock your hands around your right shin.

※ Keeping your head and shoulders on the floor, gently ease your right knee away from you, resisting with your hands.

※ Close your eyes, let go and breathe, and hold for 10 counts. Release and then repeat on the other side.

※ Complete this sequence 3 times, breathing as you work.

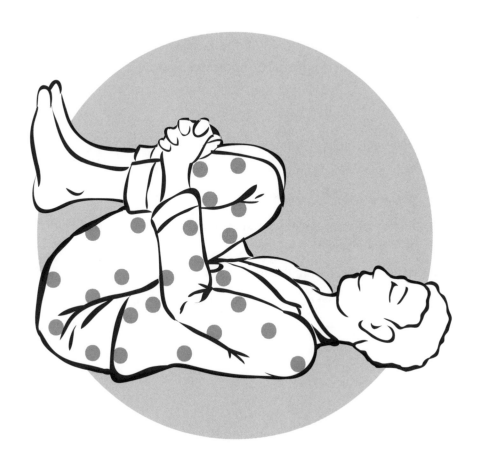

YOGABACKRUB

knee hug with strap

KNEE HUG WITH STRAP relaxes the body while providing an easy stretch for the muscles running along the spine.

you will need: *1 strap*

* Create a wide loop around your body with a fastened strap.

* Recline, positioning the strap under your lower back.

* Hug your knees through the strap and into your chest.

* Tighten the strap around your shins, gently stretching your hips. Relax your head and shoulders to the floor.

* Find a comfortable position for your arms.

* Close your eyes, let go and relax, and hold for 1 to 3 minutes.

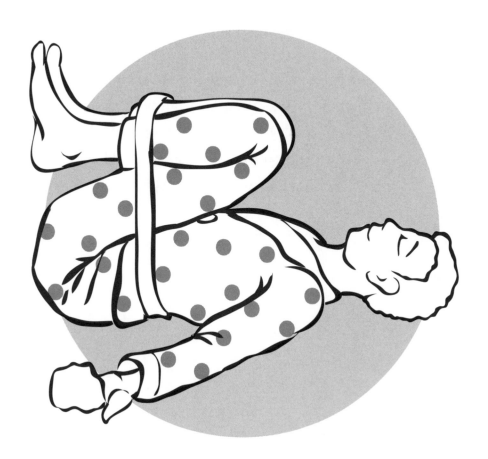

YOGABACKRUB

6

WE EAT TOO much junk and not enough vegetables. We sleep too little and overdose on caffeine. We breathe in too much exhaust and not enough oxygen. We drink sodas the size of buckets, but are dreadfully dehydrated. We skip walks outside in favor of channel surfing on the sofa. We work nonstop and ignore our health. We live lives of both excess and deprivation. Our systems are totally out of balance.

We feel sluggish, bloated and drained. Our skin breaks out, our hair falls out, our nails are brittle and weak. We are toxic. We need a YogaCleanse. Restorative yoga postures, especially twists, help the body flush toxins and waste while melting away stress, allowing us to easily let go of the hardness and tightness that often prevent our bodies from self-regulating. Restful poses also work on a deeper level, helping us get in touch with our bodies so that we become more sensitive and mindful of how we care for ourselves.

The sequence of YogaCleanse poses in this chapter will purify the body and nurture the spirit. Soon we'll notice parking our cars a little farther away from the building, just to enjoy a nice walk. Without thinking, we'll choose an orange over chips. We'll feel cleaner, leaner, and lighter. Our skin will develop a glow. Just as we understand that a plant needs just the right mix of sun and shade, just the right amount of water—not too much, not too little—we'll notice our own unique needs and begin to honor them. The result is balance.

* **half dog with strap and block**

* **standing wall twist**

* **standing wall hang**

* **shoulder-opening chair hang**

* **propped-up bridge pose**

* **prayer twist**

* **lifted twist**

* **belly-breathing rest**

* **inverted chair rest**

half dog with strap and block

HALF DOG WITH STRAP AND BLOCK warms the body, increasing circulation and respiration.

you will need: *a wall, 1 strap, 1 block*

* ✳ Measure and fasten a strap loop the width of your shoulders.

* ✳ Place the loop around your arms just above your elbows. When you straighten your arms, the strap should secure your arms at shoulder width.

* ✳ Stand facing a wall.

* ✳ Bring your fingertips to the wall, level with your hips.

* ✳ Walk backward, keeping your hands, with fingertips facing the ceiling, pressed into the wall until your feet are directly under your hips.

* ✳ Separate your feet to hip-distance apart, keeping the outer edges of your feet parallel. Place a block between your thighs.

* ✳ Your body should form a right angle, legs perpendicular to and torso and arms parallel to the floor.

* ✳ Keep your ears in line with your upper arms and firm your arms until the strap begins to feel loose.

※ Attempt to squeeze the block away from the wall causing the lower back to broaden.

※ Close your eyes, let go and breathe, and hold for 30 seconds to 2 minutes. Then walk your feet toward the wall and release.

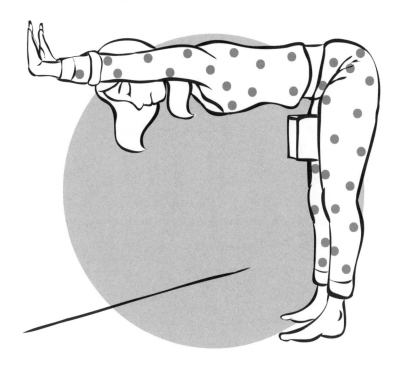

standing wall twist

STANDING WALL TWIST stimulates intestinal action by increasing blood flow to the digestive tract.

you will need: *a wall, a sturdy chair*

✳ Place a sturdy chair sideways against a wall.

✳ Stand facing the side of chair with your left side to the wall and your left foot flat on the seat.

✳ Turn your torso to face the wall, placing both hands on the wall, with your elbows bent.

✳ Pulling your shoulder blades down the back, gently ease into the twist.

✳ Close your eyes, let go and breathe, and hold for 30 seconds to 1 minute. Repeat on the other side, with the right foot on the chair and the right side of the body next to the wall.

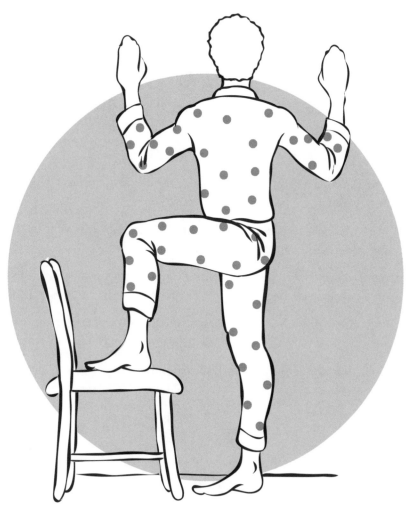

YOGA**CLEANSE**

standing wall hang

STANDING WALL HANG stretches and opens the shoulders, thus improving posture and creating an overall feeling of lightness.

you will need: *a wall*

✳ Stand facing a wall about 1 foot away, with your feet parallel and hip-distance apart.

✳ Place your palms against the wall, about 18 inches above your head, shoulder-distance apart.

✳ Gently lift your lower belly and extend your tailbone toward your heels to protect your lower back.

✳ Press into your palms, and slowly walk a little farther away from the wall, allowing your chest to melt toward the wall and stretching your shoulders.

✳ Close your eyes, let go and breathe, and hold for 30 seconds to 2 minutes.

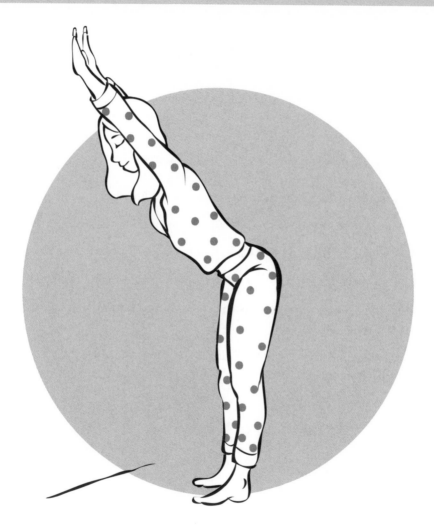

YOGACLEANSE

shoulder-opening chair hang

SHOULDER-OPENING CHAIR HANG increases opening in the shoulders and chest.

you will need: *an open-folded blanket, a sturdy chair, 1 strap, 1 block*

* Kneel on an open-folded blanket in front of a sturdy chair.

* Loop a strap just above your elbows, securing your arms at shoulder width.

* Place a block between your hands as shown.

* Place your elbows on the edge of the chair, fingertips pointing to the ceiling.

* Step your knees away from the chair until your body forms a straight line from your elbows to your hips.

* Maintain a lift in your lower belly to protect your back, and let your head relax between your upper arms to stretch your shoulders.

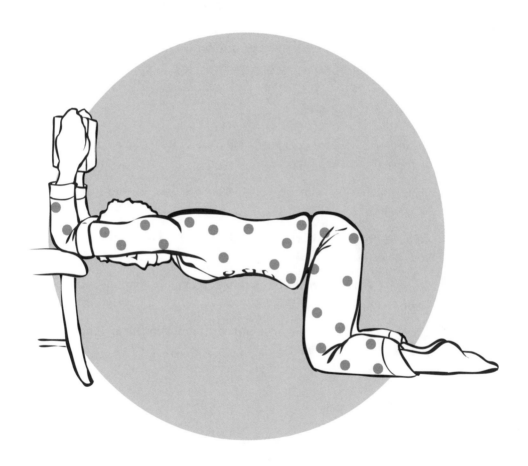

propped-up bridge pose

PROPPED-UP BRIDGE POSE relieves abdominal and menstrual cramping by gently stretching the stomach muscles.

you will need: *1 block*

* Lie on your back. Bend your knees and place your feet flat on the floor a few inches in front of your sit bones.

* Make sure the outer edges of your feet are parallel. Push into your feet and lift your hips.

* Come up on the balls of your feet and place a block directly underneath your lower back.

* Relax on the support of the block, resting your arms alongside your body, palms facing the ceiling.

* Close your eyes, let go to the support of the props and breathe, holding your pose for 1 to 3 minutes.

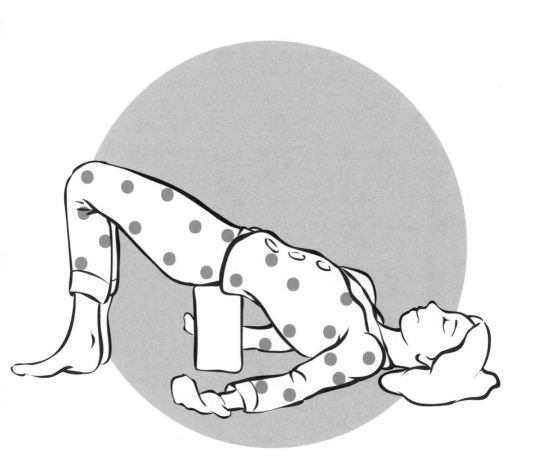

prayer twist

PRAYER TWIST gently compresses the abdomen, easing constipation and bloating.

you will need: *a sturdy chair*

* Sit in a sturdy chair with your feet flat on the floor, your feet and knees together.

* Bring your palms together at your chest.

* Hook your right elbow outside your left knee, forming a straight line from elbow to elbow.

* Avoid allowing your right knee to move forward, and gently push your left palm into your right to deepen the twist.

* Close your eyes, let go and breathe, and hold for 30 seconds to 1 minute. Repeat on the other side.

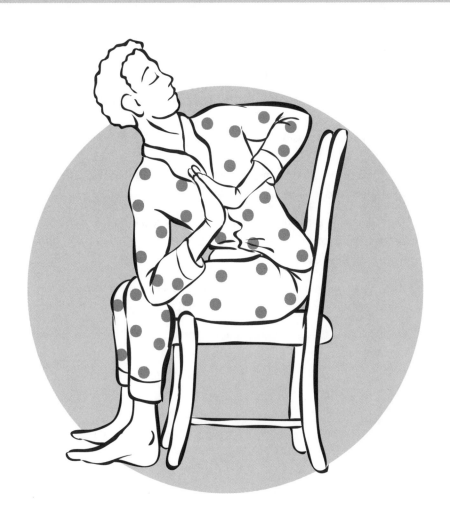

lifted twist

LIFTED TWIST stimulates the internal organs, cleansing the body.

you will need: *1 thick-rolled blanket, 1 long-folded blanket*

✳ Lie with a thick-rolled blanket supporting your middle back, with your knees bent and your feet flat on the floor.

✳ Allow both knees to drop to your left, then place a long-folded blanket between your knees and shins. The right side of your lower back will lift slightly off the blanket.

✳ Stretch your arms away from you, directly perpendicular to your body, palms facing the ceiling, and turn your chin toward your right shoulder.

✳ Close your eyes, let go and breathe, and hold for 2 to 4 minutes. Repeat on the other side.

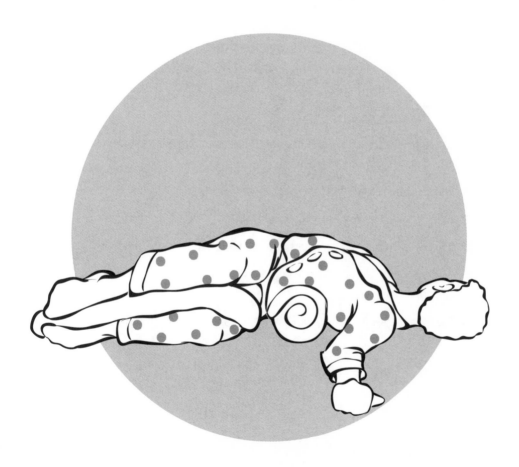

belly-breathing rest

BELLY-BREATHING REST calms the nervous system and provides a greater supply of oxygen to every cell in the body.

you will need: *1 square-folded blanket*

✳ Lie on your back with your knees bent and your feet a little wider than hip-distance apart.

✳ Place a square-folded blanket under your head.

✳ Allow your knees to drop together for support.

✳ Place your right palm on your belly and your left palm on your heart.

✳ Breathe into your palms, with your chest and belly rising and falling with each breath.

✳ Close your eyes, let go and breathe, and hold for 3 to 10 minutes.

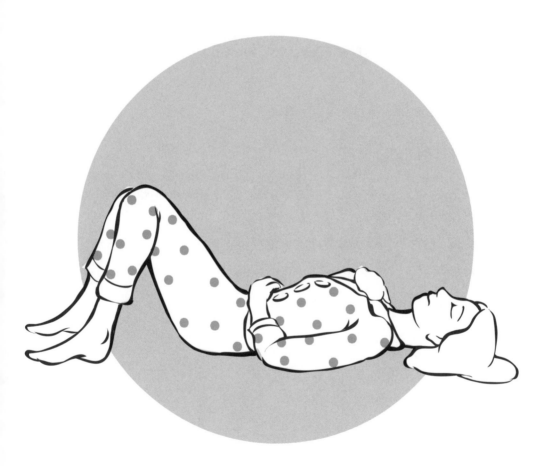

inverted chair rest

INVERTED CHAIR REST reduces stress, allowing the system to return to its natural rhythm.

you will need: *a sturdy chair, 1 open-folded blanket*

* Place an open-folded blanket on the seat of a sturdy chair.

* Lie down close to the chair, placing your calves on the seat of the chair. If necessary, add extra blankets to the seat of the chair until your bent legs form right angles.

* Allow your arms to rest alongside your body, palms facing the ceiling.

* Close your eyes, let go and breathe, and hold for 3 to 10 minutes.

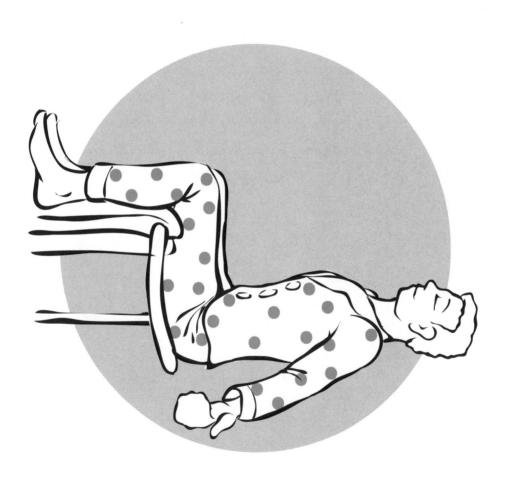

7

yogaheadacherx

SOMETIMES THEY CRAWL up the back of the neck and creep down around the forehead. Sometimes they sneak in behind the eyes. Often they push so hard on our temples, we feel like our head may explode. They appear unexpectedly and are most certainly unwelcome—awful, nagging, unpredictable headaches.

Headaches can come from a variety of sources—from tension, stress, eyestrain, air pollution, even food additives. Sometimes we get them because we have poor posture, grind our teeth, clench our jaw, or hold our breath. Muscle spasms in the shoulders, upper back, and neck restrict the flow of blood and oxygen to the brain, causing both headaches and additional stress and tension, all of which creates a downward spiral into serious pain.

Restorative yoga poses can help us relax through the pain and ease our symptoms. With regular practice, the poses in this chapter can also put an end to the vicious tension cycle and ward off future headache attacks. If your headaches persist, last longer than a couple of hours, or are accompanied by nausea, it's best to let your doctor know. Keep practicing the YogaHeadacheRx poses; consciously relax your face, shoulders, and neck throughout the day; breathe deeply; and when you least expect it, your headaches will disappear.

* **dog resting on a pillow pose**
* **head resting forward bend**
* **lazy half dog pose**
* **cross-legged chair fold**
* **angle chair fold**

* **bowing hero pose**
* **knees to forehead pose**
* **head-quieting meditation**
* **eye-soothing fold**
* **eye-wrap rest**

dog resting on a pillow pose

DOG RESTING ON A PILLOW POSE works to stretch and release the shoulder muscles, making space around the neck while providing support for the head so that the facial muscles can relax completely.

you will need: *1 bolster or 2 long-folded blankets*

✳ Kneel on all fours, with your knees directly underneath your hips—hands, knees, and feet hip-distance apart.

✳ Place a bolster and/or two long-folded blankets on the floor beneath your chest.

✳ Make sure the creases in your wrists run directly perpendicular to the length of your torso and that your arms are perfectly straight.

✳ Curl your toes under, press into your flat palms, and lift your knees up and away from the floor.

✳ Keeping your knees slightly bent, press into your hands until your body forms a straight line from your hands to your hips.

✳ Rest your head on the bolster/blankets, adjusting the height as necessary.

✳ You can work your legs toward being straight for an added stretch, if you'd like.

✳ Close your eyes, let go and breathe, and hold for 30 seconds to 2 minutes.

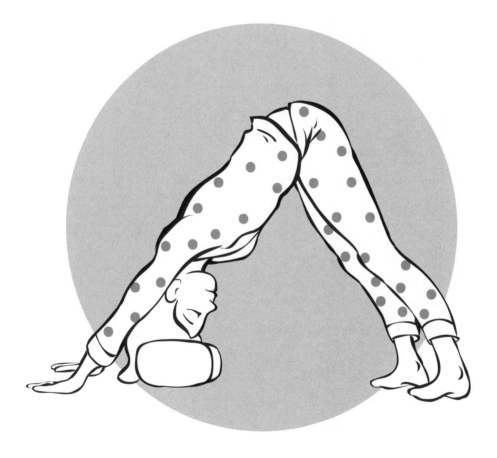

head resting forward bend

HEAD RESTING FORWARD BEND soothes the nervous system, dissolving unwanted stress.

you will need: *5 or 6 blocks*

✳ Place three or four blocks on top of each other, with an additional block to each side as shown.

✳ Stand facing the stack of blocks with your feet parallel and hip-distance apart.

✳ Fold forward, perhaps bending your knees slightly.

✳ Place the crown of your head on the stack of blocks, then place one hand on each of the side blocks.

✳ Bend your elbows to right angles, lifting your shoulders toward your waist and relaxing the facial muscles completely.

✳ Close your eyes, let go and breathe, and hold for 1 to 3 minutes.

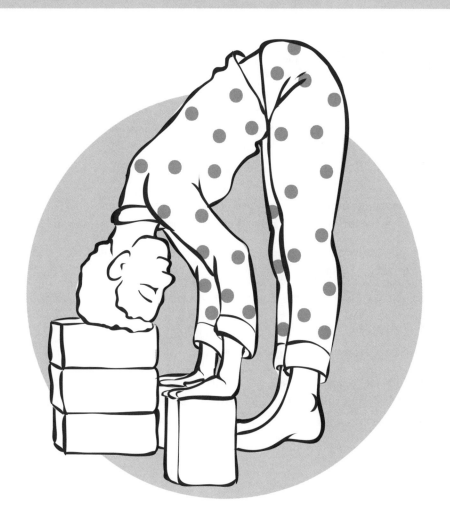

lazy half dog pose

LAZY HALF DOG POSE rests the shoulders, neck, and upper back muscles while gently stretching the muscles along the spine.

you will need: *a table, long-folded blankets or a bolster*

* Place any number of long-folded blankets or a bolster on a table (kitchen-table height), with the short end of the blankets/bolster facing you.

* Stack the props until the top of the stack is roughly the height of the very top of your thighs.

* Stand at the edge of the table, with your feet hip-distance apart and parallel.

* Fold forward, resting your torso on the props.

* Find a comfortable position for your arms.

* Turn your head to one side, close your eyes, let go and breathe, and hold for 2 to 5 minutes, turning your head to the other side halfway through the hold.

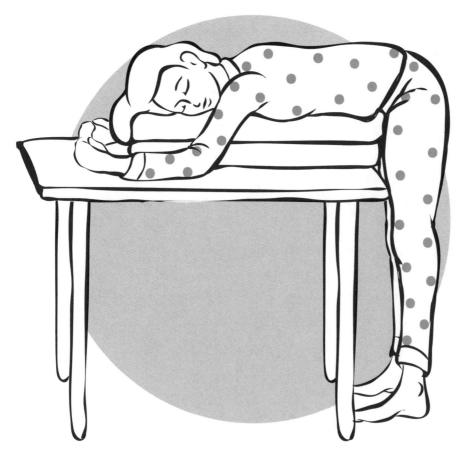

cross-legged chair fold

CROSS-LEGGED CHAIR FOLD is very calming, allowing the body to naturally release.

you will need: *1 long-folded blanket, a sturdy chair, 1 square-folded blanket*

- ✳ Place a long-folded blanket over the seat of a sturdy chair.

- ✳ Sit facing the chair in a comfortable cross-legged position, with your hips supported by a square-folded blanket.

- ✳ Gently fold forward, resting your forehead on the blanket covering the seat of the chair.

- ✳ Fold your arms onto the seat of the chair as well.

- ✳ Close your eyes, let go of your shoulders and breathe, and hold for 2 to 5 minutes, switching the crossing of your legs halfway through the hold.

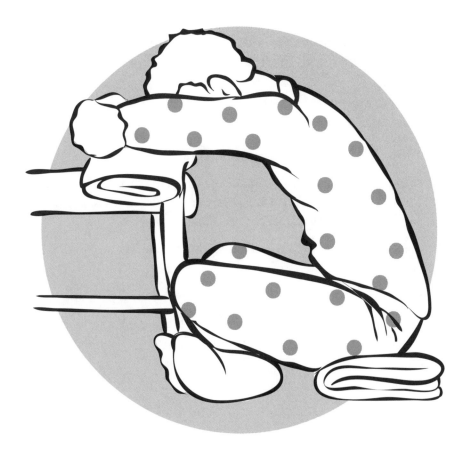

angle chair fold

ANGLE CHAIR FOLD provides a calming way to stretch the inner thighs and hips as you relax into the fold.

you will need: *1 long-folded blanket, a sturdy chair, 1 square-folded blanket, 1 or 2 blocks (optional)*

✳ Place a long-folded blanket over the seat of a sturdy chair.

✳ Sit on a square-folded blanket, facing the seat of the chair, with the soles of your feet together, heels 6 to 12 inches from you. You can support your knees with blocks if you'd like.

✳ Gently fold forward, resting your forehead on the blanket covering the seat of the chair.

✳ Fold your arms onto the seat of the chair as well.

✳ Close your eyes, let go of your shoulders and breathe, and hold for 2 to 5 minutes.

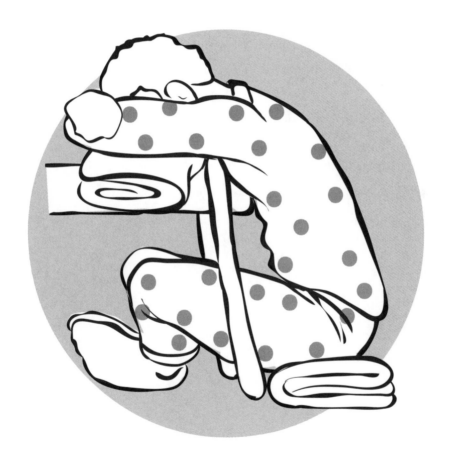

bowing hero pose

BOWING HERO POSE improves circulation.

you will need: *2 thick-rolled blankets*

* Kneel with your knees touching and your feet a little wider than hip-distance apart.

* Place a thick-rolled blanket on top of your calves and sit on it.

* Place another thick-rolled blanket in front of you.

* Bow forward from the hips, resting your head and arms on the blanket. Your spine will be in a slight natural curve.

* Close your eyes, let go and breathe, and hold for 1 to 3 minutes.

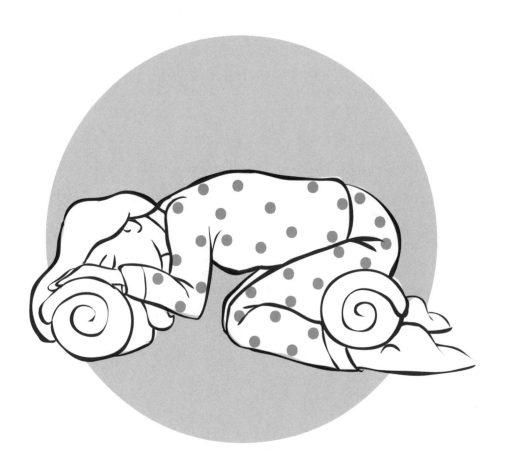

knees to forehead pose

KNEES TO FOREHEAD POSE can be slightly precarious at first. Take your time to find your balance, and allow the gentle pressure of your knees to melt away headache pain.

you will need: *1 thick-rolled blanket*

* Lie down with a thick-rolled blanket under your middle back.

* With your hands pressing into the floor for leverage, sweep your legs over your head and rest your knees on your forehead.

* Interlock your hands behind you on top of the blanket.

* Bend your knees so the tops of your knees are resting on your forehead and your heels are melting toward your buttocks.

* Close your eyes, let go and breathe, and hold for 30 seconds to 1 minute.

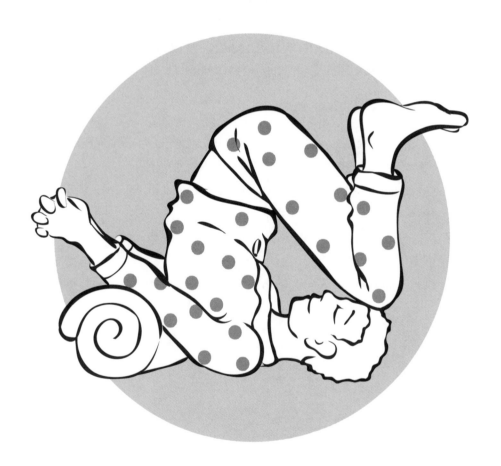

head-quieting meditation

HEAD-QUIETING MEDITATION focuses on the nervous system. Breathing fully and smoothly will pacify any residual stress.

you will need: *a wall, 1 blanket or bolster*

* Sit with your back against a wall in a comfortable cross-legged position, with your hips supported by a blanket or a bolster.

* Straighten your arms, bringing the backs of your hands to rest on your knees.

* Relax your shoulders, and gently bring together the thumb and middle finger of each hand.

* Close your eyes, let go, and internally watch your breath for at least 5 minutes.

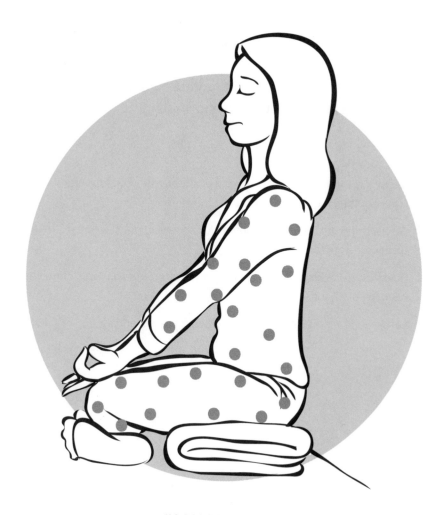

eye-soothing fold

EYE-SOOTHING FOLD will provide gentle support and pressure for your head while blocking out agitating light.

you will need: *1 square-folded blanket or 1 bolster*

❋ Begin in a comfortable cross-legged position, with your hips elevated by a square-folded blanket or bolster.

❋ Gently bring the heels of your hands up to cover your closed eyes, palms resting on your forehead.

❋ Bow forward from your hips, head approaching your lap, supporting your head in your hands.

❋ Let go and breathe, holding this position for 30 seconds.

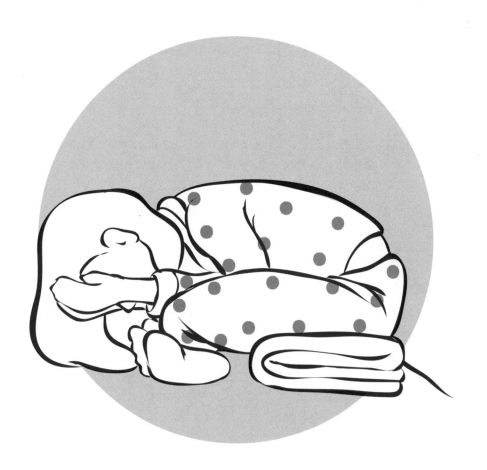

eye-wrap rest

EYE-WRAP REST will provide just the escape and soothing quiet needed to relieve your headache.

you will need: *2 open-folded blankets, 1 long-folded blanket, 1 towel or cloth*

* Create an incline with two open-folded blankets and one long-folded blanket so that the lower "step" will support your calves, and the upper "step" will support your feet.

* Wrap a towel or cloth around your head, covering your eyes to block the light completely.

* Lie down with your lower legs supported by the blankets.

* Position your arms alongside your body with the palms facing the ceiling.

* Close your eyes, let go of your jaw and facial muscles, breathe deeply, and hold for 5 to 10 minutes.

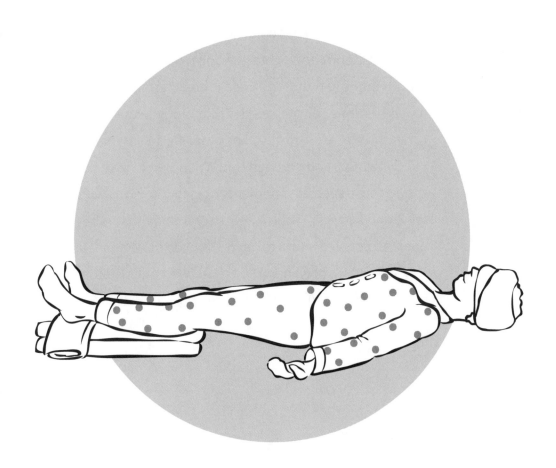

8

yogabreak

YOU KNOW HOW it is. Phones ring off the hook, deadlines loom, bosses breathe down our necks, and e-mails mount into the hundreds. We eat breakfast in our cars and lunch or dinner at our desks. Technology keeps speeding up and we're expected to keep up. We feel overworked, overwhelmed, and stressed out. When we do take five, we spend those precious moments dosing ourselves with caffeine and sugar. We futilely reach for energy that is beyond our grasp, only to return to our desks even more drained, and worse—totally bewildered because we conned ourselves into thinking we were taking a break.

Little pauses for yoga throughout the day can help slow our racing hearts, and deep breathing will ease our tender nerves. Many of the YogaBreak poses in this chapter can be done at your desk or in your office, some while on the phone, and none require special props. A few are even discreet enough to be practiced during long meetings or conferences. Taking just a few YogaBreaks a day will help us let go of tension before it turns into stress. We'll be able to channel more energy into our work, and our bosses will be thrilled with our greater productivity. Who knows, one day we might even jump up and say, "Yay ... It's Monday!"

* **steering wheel twist**

* **elevator forward bend**

* **neck and wrist rolls**

* **desk chair fold**

* **twist and relax pose**

* **office ankle to knee pose**

* **stiff legs stretch**

* **anti-slouch wall hang**

* **easy boat pose**

* **mini yoganap**

steering wheel twist

Before you get out of the car in the morning and face your day, take a quick twist. THE STEERING WHEEL TWIST wakes up and stretches your spine.

✳ While parked, hold your steering wheel at the 10 and 2 o'clock positions, lift your chest and twist your upper torso.

✳ Close your eyes, let go and breathe deeply, holding your position on each side for a few breaths.

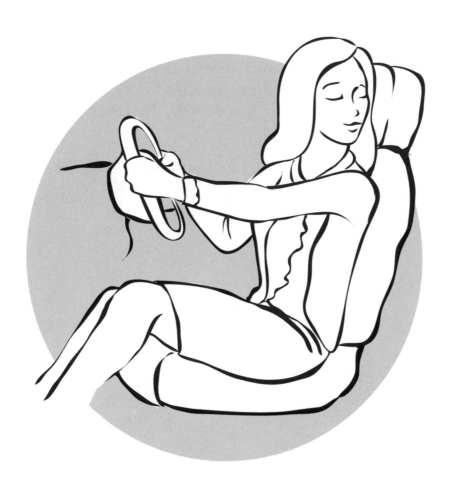

elevator forward bend

When you find yourself alone in the elevator, instead of watching the numbers above you, use the time wisely by doing the ELEVATOR FORWARD BEND. This stretch lengthens your back and eases neck and shoulder strain.

* Rest your hips on the wall and fold forward. Really let your head and neck go.

* Close your eyes, let go and breathe, and hold till you reach your destination. Be sure to roll up slowly.

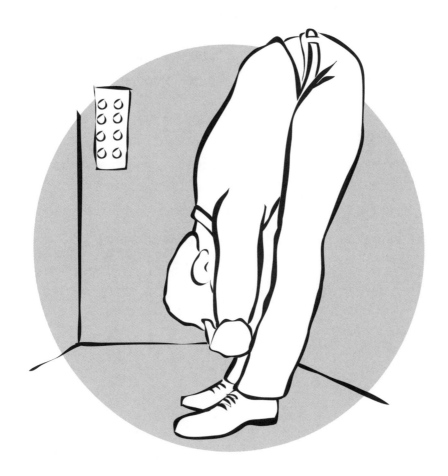

YOGABREAK

neck and wrist rolls

NECK AND WRIST ROLLS massage away the kinks and stiffness that come from working at a desk or computer for long periods.

✳ Roll away tension by making gentle circles with your head and hands with gently curved fingers.

✳ Make large rolls with your neck, dropping your chin all the way to your chest and trying to touch your shoulder with your ear.

✳ Try rolling your neck to the right for a few circles and then to the left.

✳ Try varying the size of the wrist circles and finish by stretching through your fingers.

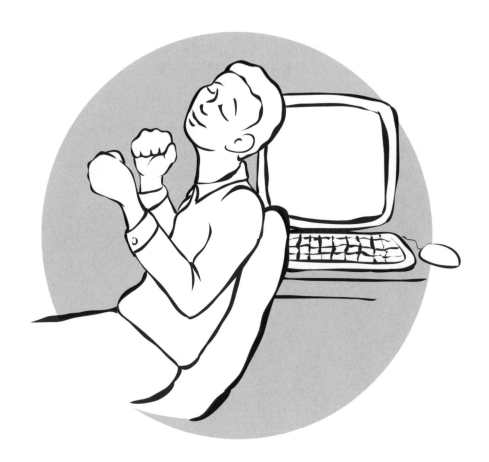

YOGABREAK

desk chair fold

If your hips feel tight from sitting a lot, the DESK CHAIR FOLD can bring relief. It releases your lower back and brings flexibility into your hip joints.

✳ Fold forward from the hips, folding between wide knees and feet, letting your head and arms dangle.

✳ Close your eyes, let go and breathe, and hold for about a minute.

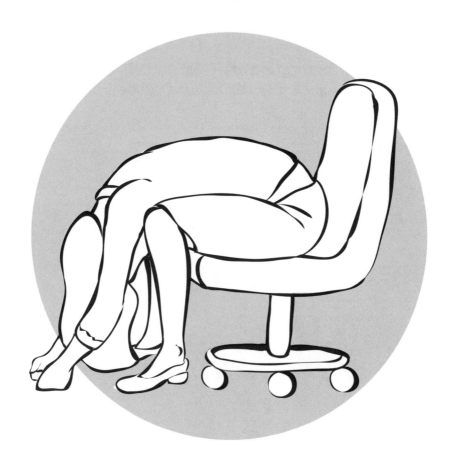

twist and relax pose

A tired, aching back is no surprise at the office, and there's no better way to relieve midday back pain then the TWIST AND RELAX POSE. It's a perfect little pick-me-up anytime your back feels crunched and achy.

※ Stand in back of your chair. Grab the back of it, then lift your chest and twist from your waist.

※ Close your eyes, let go and breathe, and hold for 30 seconds.

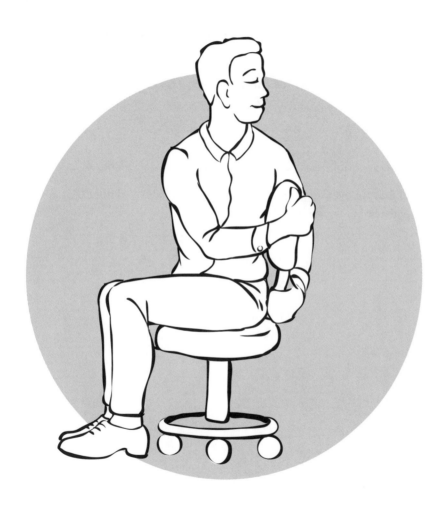

office ankle to knee pose

Even in a meeting there's time for yoga! The OFFICE ANKLE TO KNEE POSE opens and relaxes your hips. But only you will know that you're taking a YogaBreak.

* Cross your right ankle over your left knee and let your knee drop.

* Close your eyes, let go and breathe, and hold for one minute. Then repeat with left ankle over right knee.

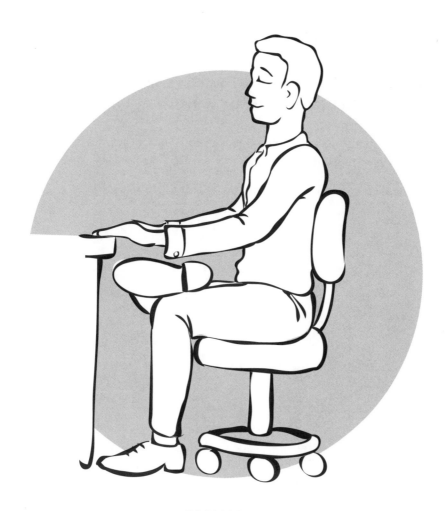

stiff-legs stretch

Sitting for hours can wreak wreak havoc on your hamstrings. The STIFF-LEGS STRETCH relieves hamstring tightness.

✳ Scoot to the edge of your chair, stretch your legs out straight in front of you, and bend forward from the hips.

✳ Close your eyes, let go and breathe, and hold for 30 seconds.

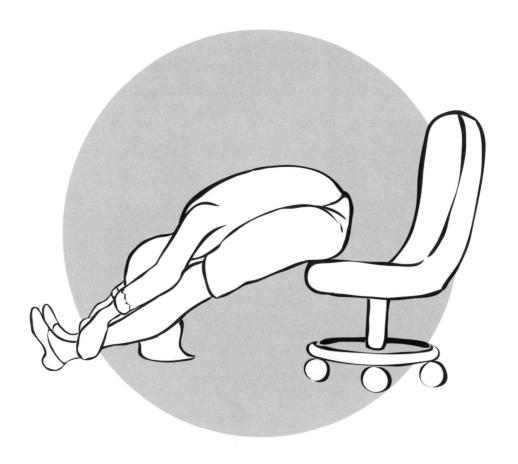

anti-slouch wall hang

Do you find yourself hunched over your desk or keyboard all day? The ANTI-SLOUCH WALL HANG stretches your shoulders and improves your posture—you'll stand taller, feel more awake, and have more confidence.

✳ Walk your hands up a wall until they are about 18 inches above your head.

✳ Step back from the wall and hang, stretching your shoulders.

✳ Close your eyes, feel the sensation, and breathe for one minute.

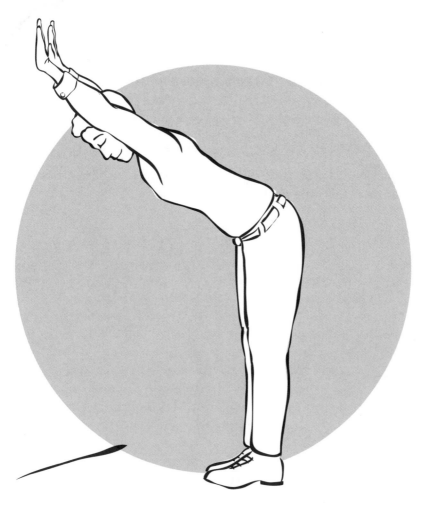

YOGABREAK

easy boat pose

EASY BOAT POSE is just the rest you need for aching feet and legs.

* Relax, take your shoes off! Sit at your desk and put your feet up!

* Lean your head back, close your eyes, and let go and breathe.

* Imagine you're on a tropical beach or standing in an open meadow—anyplace that makes you feel calm!

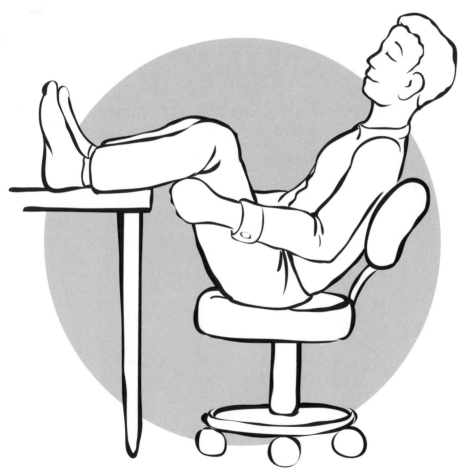

YOGABREAK

mini yoganap

There's always time for a YOGANAP. Taking a brief rest can energize your body and mind for the rest of the day.

* Rest your forehead on your desk, propped on folded forearms. (You might even want to keep a little pillow at the office.)

* Set your computer timer so you'll be able to rest completely without worry.

* Close your eyes! Breathe! Let go! Rest completely!

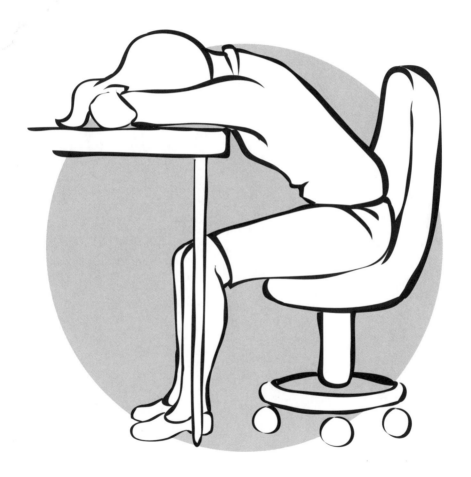